MAX O$_2$

Also by **Health For Life**:

- **Legendary Abs II**

- **Beyond Legendary Abs**

- **Power ForeArms!**

- **T.N.T.—Total Neck & Traps**

- **Maximum Calves**

- **The Human Fuel Handbook**
  Nutrition for Peak Athletic Performance

- **The *Health For Life* Training Advisor**

- **SynerStretch:** For Whole Body Flexibility

- **Minimizing Reflex and Reaction Time**

- **Amino Acids & Other Ergogenic Aids**

- **Explosive Power**
  Plyometrics for Bodybuilders, Martial Artists, and Other Athletes

- **Secrets of Advanced Bodybuilders**
  A manual of synergistic weight training for the whole body

ISBN 0-944831-30-3
Library of Congress Catalog Card Number: 93-73083

Health For Life
8033 Sunset Blvd., Suite 483 — Los Angeles, CA 90046 — (310) 306-0777

1 2 3 4 5 6 7 8 9

MAX O$_2$

THE COMPLETE GUIDE TO SYNERGISTIC AEROBIC TRAINING

Jerry Robinson
Frank Carrino

Health For Life

Pour Tonton

To Sandy and Courtney
for their inspiration, love, and support

CREDITS AND ACKNOWLEDGMENTS

Special thanks to
Ed Derse, Lance Laterza,
Robert Miller, Brian Shiers,
and Dr. Eric Sternlicht for
their guidance and
suggestions during
the development of
Max O2

Edited by Robert Miller
Book design and
illustration by
Irene DiConti McKinniss
Additional artwork
by Karl Shields
Typesetting by Jack Hazelton

CONTENTS

PART TWO — TRAINING

PART THREE — SUPPORT

APPENDIX

INTRODUCTION

INTRODUCTION

For many years, it's been *all quiet on the aerobic front*—there haven't been any changes in basic aerobic training recommendations. In fact, you can probably reel off the generic fitness program in your sleep...

- Jog, swim, climb stairs, or do some other whole-body activity at a sweat-inducing pace
- Work out 3 to 4 times per week
- Do 20 to 40 minutes per session

If you like to run the Ironman or compete in one of the other elite endurance torture-fests, your program may have been a bit more complicated. But, basically, aerobic training has always boiled down to the same thing—increasing the body's capacity to absorb, transport, and use oxygen in producing muscular energy for prolonged activity. Physiologists describe this capacity in terms of the largest volume of oxygen your body can use during exercise—a value called your **VO2 max**.

Well, times are changing! New research shows that our old aerobics model has a big piece missing. That piece is called the **lactate threshold**, and it's *at least* as important as VO2 max in determining your aerobic fitness. Unlike VO2 max, which is determined by the body's *overall* ability to absorb and transport oxygen, your lactate threshold is influenced by a *local* factor: the endurance of the specific muscles involved in an exercise.

It's the lactate threshold behind the following surprising effect: If you train one group of people on a treadmill and another group on a rowing machine, the group that *trained* on the treadmill will show a significant improvement in VO_2 max when *tested* on a treadmill *but little improvement when tested on a rower!* Similarly, the group that trained on a rowing machine will show significant improvement when tested on a rowing machine but little improvement when tested on a treadmill.

This connection between training exercise and testing exercise shows that aerobic capacity is much more closely linked to the endurance of specific muscles than we previously thought. And *that* means that if aerobic training is going to be effective, **it *can't* just target VO_2 max, as it has in the past. It must *also* target the lactate threshold.** Each requires its own kind of training.

Furthermore, as we'll see, even subtly different training goals may require very different ratios of VO_2 max to lactate threshold work. Take two people both trying to lose weight— a bodybuilder and someone just carrying a few extra pounds. If the bodybuilder uses the overweight person's ideal aerobic program, he or she may drop *muscle* as well as fat. And if the overweight person tries the bodybuilder's ideal pre-contest fat-loss program, he or she won't shed the extra pounds nearly as fast as possible. Not the desired result in either case! (And no, this isn't just a matter of training at different intensities.)

So what's the best way to improve VO_2 max *and* your lactate threshold, and how do you balance these two aspects of training to reach different goals? We have to cover some ground to explain. Don't worry. It isn't important to memorize all the gory physiological details. What *is* important is understanding how your body produces energy—both with oxygen and without it. That's the focus of the upcoming *Foundation* section.

Then, in the *Training* section, we'll explore the ultimate regimens to get fit, hit low bodyfat levels for a bodybuilding contest, generally lose weight, and even get ready for marathons and other endurance events. You'll also find special "how-to" chapters here on a pair of activities ideal for lactate-threshold training: slideboarding and jumping rope.

Finally, in the *Support* section, we'll look at peripheral topics—nutrition for optimum aerobic performance, sports drinks, ergogenic aids, and so on.

So let's go to it! Get set for a remarkable new way of looking at aerobic training.

❖   ❖   ❖

PART ONE

Foundation

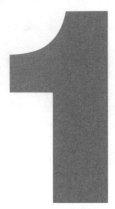

HEART, LUNGS, & BLOOD

The six short chapters in this section lay the groundwork for the training programs to come. They're like pieces of a puzzle. Each is complete in its own right, but you may not immediately see how they fit together. Fear not! Just like the last page of a Sherlock Holmes story, Chapter 7 will explain all. We begin at the beginning, with the air you breathe....

THE CARDIOVASCULAR SYSTEM

Muscles produce energy by different processes. Some involve oxygen; some don't. Those that do we call **aerobic**, literally meaning *with oxygen*. Those that don't, we call *an***aerobic**, which means *without oxygen*.

For aerobic energy production to take place, oxygen first has to get to the muscles. It does that via the **cardiovascular system**—the heart, lungs, and the network of vessels that route blood through the body.* To get a clear picture of how the cardiovascular system works, let's follow a few molecules of oxygen from air to muscle.

Cardio means heart; *vascular* refers to the the vessels that transport blood. So strictly speaking, the term *cardiovascular* doesn't include the lungs. In fact, none of the terms usually used to refer to the combination of heart, lungs, and circulatory system (*cardiovascular*, *cardiorespiratory*, and the academically preferred *circulo-respiratory*) actually reference all three. But through common usage, both *cardiovascular* and *cardiorespiratory* have come to.

I t's a nice day out, so you decide to take a walk. As you stride briskly down the sidewalk, a group of muscles in your chest, called the **inspiratory muscles**, expand your rib cage. Like spreading the handles on a bellows, this decreases the pressure in your chest and air rushes in to fill the available space.

The air enters through your nose, where it's moistened, filtered, and warmed to body temperature (or cooled, if you live in the Sahara desert). All this processing ensures that any air you breathe is in a nice palatable condition by the time it passes through your nasal cavities. From there, it flows on to your pharynx, larynx, and trachea (also known as the windpipe), finally entering the lungs through large tubes called **bronchii** (Fig. 1).

IN THE LUNGS

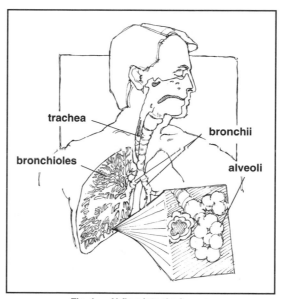

Fig. 1 — Airflow into the Lungs

The bronchii divide into smaller tubes, called **bronchioles**. These divide into yet smaller tubes...which divide into yet smaller tubes...and on and on until the air (containing our few oxygen molecules) finally ends up in clusters of tiny microscopic sacs called **alveoli**. Within the alveoli, the actual extraction of oxygen from the air takes place, like this: Part of each alveoli faces into the lungs, bringing it into contact with the air you just inhaled. Another part faces out, bringing it into contact with an intricate network of blood vessels that suffuse lung tissue. Through a process called **diffusion**, each alveoli extracts oxygen from the air and passes it through the membrane of the lungs, depositing it neatly in the bloodstream (Fig. 2).

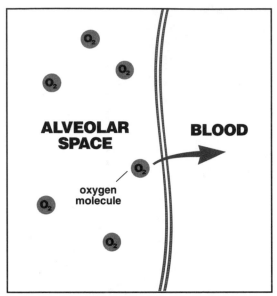

Fig. 2 — Oxygen Diffusing into the Blood Stream

IN THE BLOOD

The oxygen molecules we're tracking flow within the blood through a vast network of vessels in your body, ranging in size from the half-inch aorta, the artery serving as a blood-transport super-highway out of the heart, to the microscopic capillaries—over 40 billion of them—that spread throughout the body's tissues.

As we just said, a whole network of those capillaries come into contact with alveoli in the lungs. The alveoli act just like New York subway stations (without the muggers), providing a two-way platform where oxygen, extracted from the air you breathe, enters the bloodstream; and carbon dioxide, one of the waste products of aerobic energy production, leaves the bloodstream enroute to being exhaled.

If the alveoli are the subway *stations*, then your blood is one gigantic subway *train*, transporting nutrients to all parts of the body.

Oxygen gets special treatment. Special cells in the blood—**red blood cells**, or **erythrocytes**—act as oxygen subway *cars*, and special molecules within the red blood cells, **hemoglobin** molecules, act as the oxygen subway car *seats*. When the alveoli extract oxygen out of the air in the lungs, it passes through the capillary walls into the hemoglobin molecules within the red blood cells (Fig. 3).

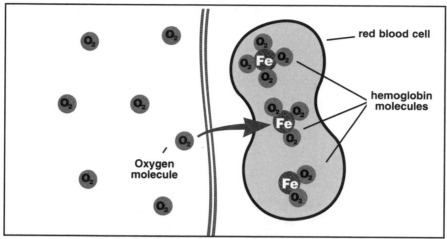

Fig. 3 — An Oxygen Molecule Entering a Red Blood Cell and Attaching to a Hemoglobin Molecule

Every single hemoglobin molecule can seat four oxygen molecules. Since there are about 280 million hemoglobin molecules per red blood cell, each red blood cell can transport more than a billion molecules of oxygen!

So, our oxygen molecules—along with many, many others—move from the lungs to the blood, specifically to the hemoglobin molecules, in which they are whisked off to the muscles.

THROUGH THE HEART

Subway trains need engines. Yours is the heart. This hollow, fist-sized muscle lies in the center of your chest (slightly offset to the left), nestled between the lungs in an area called the **mediastinum**. The heart pumps about 80 million gallons of blood through your circulatory system during your lifetime. Depending on the body's demand, it can push out from 5 to 35 liters per minute. That's 5.2 to 37 quarts. Since the amount of oxygen that reaches your muscles depends a lot on how much and how fast your blood gets circulated, **cardiac output** has a major effect on your aerobic capacity.

Cardiac output depends on two things: **stroke volume** and **frequency**.

Stroke volume is just what it sounds like—the amount of blood pumped out of the heart in a single stroke. *Frequency* is the number of strokes per minute—better known as your **heart rate**. Multiply stroke volume times frequency and you have the total amount of blood the heart pumps per minute.

VO_2 max training increases both components of cardiac output: it increases the amount of blood pumped per stroke, and it allows you to work safely at a heart rate closer to your maximum heart rate. More on that later when we talk in detail about how to get the greatest effect from that part of your aerobic training.

AT THE MUSCLES

So—our oxygen molecules, which start out as one of the three main components of the air you breathe, flow into your lungs. There, the alveoli separate out the O_2 and pass it, by diffusion, to the hemoglobin molecules in the blood. The blood flows through the heart, which pumps it out to the muscles where it's ready to be used in any of several aerobic energy production processes. In the next chapter, we'll begin looking at some of those energy production processes, both aerobic and not.

❖ ❖ ❖

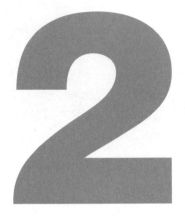

ATP, CARBOHYDRATE, FAT, & PROTEIN

There are two ways to explore the processes your body uses to produce energy. You can start with the *fuels* involved. This approach points the way toward the diet that promotes optimum aerobic performance (and, as it turns out, maximum weight loss, too). Or you can start with the circumstances under which each energy process makes its greatest contribution. This leads (via a somewhat circuitous route through VO$_2$ max and the lactate threshold) to the formula for optimum aerobic training.

First things first: Let's look at the fuels.

ATP

Pick up any article on sports nutrition, and you'll probably read something to the effect that your body "burns" carbohydrate, fat, or protein to produce energy. Actually, statements like that are misleading. Although carbohydrate, fat, and protein all *participate* in various energy-production processes, what really gets "burned" is something called **ATP**.

ATP—**A**denosine **TriP**hosphate—is a special molecule whose structure allows it to store a lot of energy. It's like a compressed spring. Break the bonds that hold an ATP molecule together and you release the energy, just like letting the spring go. *Energy from ATP breakdown directly fuels every physiological* *process in your body.* Without ATP, none of those processes could take place.

At any time, though, you only have about 3 ounces of ATP distributed throughout your cells. That's roughly enough to fuel a 6-second all-out sprint. So how can you run an 8-second sprint? Or a 400 meter? Or a marathon? Enter the other fuels. Through several physiological processes, carbohydrate, fat, and protein continuously participate in the creation of new ATP.

Let's see how this works.

CARBOHYDRATE

Thanks to whatever pasta, bread, or other carbohydrates you've eaten over the past few days, you now have about 375 to 475 grams' worth of carbs stored in your body.

- Roughly 325 grams are stored as **glycogen**, a simple sugar, in your muscles.
- Another 90 to 110 grams are stored, also as glycogen, in your liver.
- The remaining 15 to 20 grams are floating around as **glucose** in your blood.

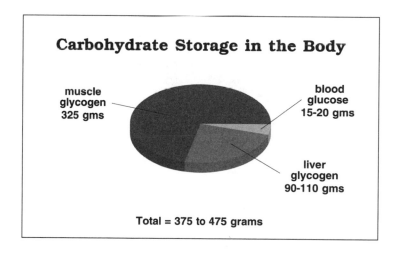

Carbohydrate Storage in the Body

muscle glycogen 325 gms

blood glucose 15-20 gms

liver glycogen 90-110 gms

Total = 375 to 475 grams

Each of those grams of carbohydrate contains 4 calories of energy, which means you have roughly 1500 to 2000 calories available from your carb stores, or about enough to power a 20-mile run. If you eat a high-carb diet for a few days, you can double that—to a maximum of about 15 grams per kilogram of bodyweight (about 1100 grams for the average male adult).

Aerobic & Anaerobic Glycolysis

All that carbohydrate can be used to produce new ATP. In fact, all that carbohydrate can be used to produce new ATP both in the presence *and absence* of oxygen. If there's enough oxygen around to produce ATP from carbohydrate aerobically (with oxygen), you get a lot of ATP. For every molecule of glucose you put in, you get **36** molecules of ATP out, via a process called **aerobic glycolysis**. If, on the other hand, there isn't enough oxygen around and the ATP is produced from carbohydrate *anaerobically* (without oxygen), the yield isn't so great. For each molecule of glucose you put in, you only get **2** molecules of ATP out, via a process called *anaerobic* **glycolysis**.

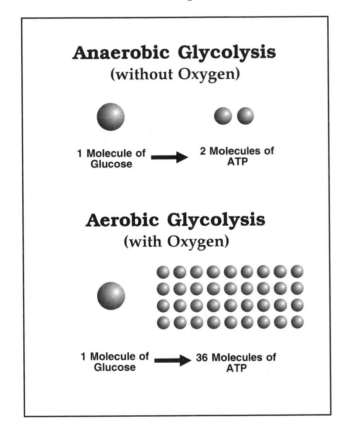

When you get up out of your chair and begin running, cycling, or swimming, *anaerobic* glycolysis provides the ATP for most of the energy. It remains the primary ATP source for about 3 to 5 minutes—the time it takes for your cardiovascular system to get up to speed.

Then, for the next 20 minutes, *aerobic* glycolysis provides about 40% to 50% of the ATP for energy. Beyond that point, carbohydrate contribution falls until, at the 4-hour point, aerobic glycolysis may be meeting just 5% of the total energy demands.

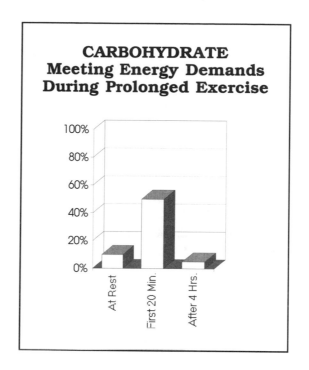

CARBOHYDRATE
Meeting Energy Demands
During Prolonged Exercise

FAT

Let's not belabor where your body gets its fat stores. Suffice it to say that, at 9 calories per gram, a gram of fat contains more than twice the potential energy of a gram of carbohydrate. Figure the average well-nourished adult male carries about 15% of his weight in fat. That means he's got about 100,000 available calories in his fat stores—or enough to keep him running for 119 hours! Women tend to carry slightly more fat than men, so most have even *more* potential energy in their fat stores. Clearly, energy from fat is *not* the limiting factor during most endurance events.

Fat participates in energy production in two ways: First, a small part of each fat molecule can be converted anaerobically to glucose. This, in turn, can be dumped into the carbohydrate-burning processes we discussed above to produce ATP. Second—and much more significant—in the presence of enough oxygen, a different part of that single fat molecule can be processed to yield a whopping 441 molecules of ATP! Compare that to the relatively puny 36 ATP you can get from a molecule of carbohydrate.

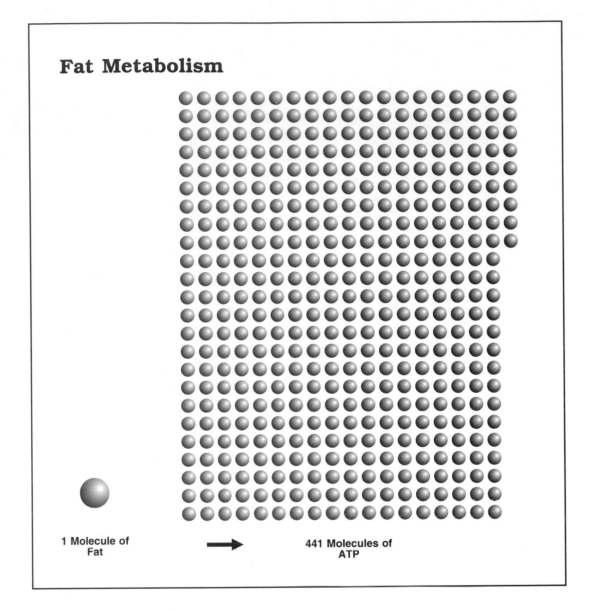

Fat Metabolism

1 Molecule of Fat → **441 Molecules of ATP**

Fat metabolism provides upwards of 90% of the ATP you need at rest. It's responsible for about 50% to 60% of the ATP required during the first 20 minutes of submaximal exercise. And that rises to about 80% after 4 hours of continuous training.

One very important note we'll return to later: Despite the prodigious amounts of energy you can get from fat metabolism, it has a major limitation—*fat can only be used to produce energy in the presence of carbohydrate (and oxygen).* As exercise physiologists McArdle, Katch, and Katch put it, "fats burn in a carbohydrate flame." So once you've depleted your carbohydrate stores, muscular energy production must fall off.

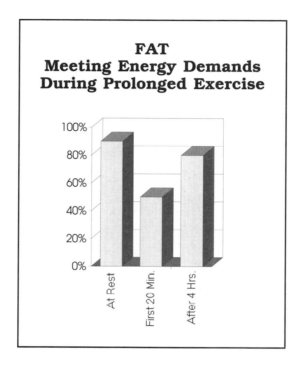

FAT
Meeting Energy Demands
During Prolonged Exercise

PROTEIN

So, you say, you had a great steak last night? The main function of dietary protein is to supply amino acids for a myriad of bodily functions that need them. But protein also figures into ATP production. Like fat, amino acids can be broken down and a certain part of them can be converted to glucose. That glucose can then be used by either aerobic or anaerobic glycolysis to produce ATP. Amino acids can contribute to ATP production in other ways as well.

Protein metabolism provides about 2% to 5% of the ATP you need at rest. After 4 hours of continuous light exercise, that figure rises to 10% to 15%.

Research shows that the more severe the exercise, the greater the percentage of energy supplied by protein breakdown. This is not a good thing. Protein for use in energy production comes from amino acids in your blood and from the degradation of tissues containing protein—*including lean muscle*. Now, most of the athletes we know would rather their structural protein molecules stay right where they are, in their muscles. Luckily, you can limit the degree to which protein degradation fuels muscular energy production by doing two things: eating a high-carbohydrate diet and maintaining an adequate caloric intake. Both exert a **protein sparing effect**, decreasing protein's tumble into energy-production pathways.

No matter what you do, though, you can't eliminate the utilization of protein for energy production entirely.

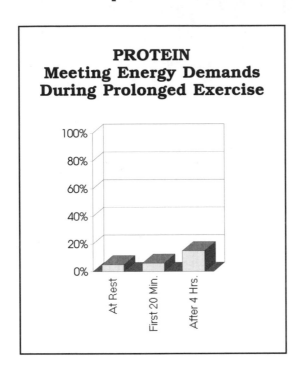

PROTEIN
Meeting Energy Demands
During Prolonged Exercise

THE POINT

Protein, carbohydrate, and fat all participate in the making of new ATP via various energy production processes. Depending on your training goal, you may wish you could shift the balance of those processes to favor the metabolism of one or another of the macronutrients. For example, if you're a bodybuilder, you may wish you could encourage more fat- and carbohydrate-burning—and less protein-degradation—during your workouts.

To a certain extent, you can. The balance of macronutrients used for energy during exercise depends on three things:

■ The length of your workout
■ The severity of your workout
■ Your diet

In a nutshell, the longer you train, the more fat burned; the higher the intensity, the more carbs burned; and the higher your carb intake, the more carbs and the less protein burned. We'll talk more in forthcoming chapters about manipulating both diet and exercise to control the storage and use of the macronutrients.

❖   ❖   ❖

Energy, Intensity, & Duration

In the last chapter, we looked at energy production from the standpoint of the fuels involved. Now we're going to take the second approach and see which circumstances favor which energy process. To keep things simple, let's distill all the processes we've covered into a few catchall groups.

There are basically three forms of energy production:

■ the **direct use of** *already available* **ATP**

■ **anaerobic processes**, such as anaerobic glycolysis, which provide *some* additional ATP. (main raw fuel: carbohydrates) ...and...

■ **aerobic processes**, such as aerobic glycolysis, which provide a *lot* of additional ATP. (raw fuels: carbohydrates, *plus* fat and protein)

All three forms supply energy continuously. Which one takes the lead depends on the **intensity** and **duration** of activity.

VERY HIGH INTENSITY, VERY SHORT DURATION

When you take off on a sprint, the demand for more energy rises suddenly—so suddenly, in fact, that your cardiovascular system can't supply additional oxygen for aerobic energy production fast enough to meet the need. At first, there isn't even time to get anaerobic glycolysis into the act.

There's only time for one thing—the direct breakdown of stored ATP.*

In general, direct ATP breakdown provides the instantaneous energy for transitions to higher activity levels—such as going from sitting to walking, or from jogging to sprinting. It's also your main source for bursts of maximum effort, such as running a 50-yard dash, doing a single power-clean, or throwing a punch.

ATP breakdown is sometimes called the *immediate* **energy source**.

The *Immediate* Energy Source

Provides energy for...

- transitions to higher activity levels
- burst of maximum effort

Remember that the direct ATP pathway can max out in as little as 6 seconds. Well, 6 seconds into an all-out sprint, the cardiovascular system still isn't up to speed. That means aerobic energy production isn't yet available; the demand has

HIGH INTENSITY, SHORT DURATION

---

*Actually, the direct breakdown of ATP gets a bit of help from another process. There's a substance within muscle cells, called CP, short for *creatine phosphate*. Like ATP, CP is a high-energy molecule. Like ATP, when you break apart a CP molecule, energy is released that can be used to power metabolic processes.

You have about three times as much CP in each muscle cell as ATP. Any time you step up activity (and thus your energy demands) so quickly that none of the carbohydrate-, fat-, or protein-using pathways can contribute, direct ATP breakdown supplies the energy, with limited new ATP synthesis fueled by the breakdown of CP.

to be met anaerobically. Anaerobic glycolysis takes the lead as direct ATP breakdown slows.

Often referred to as the *short-term* **energy source**, anaerobic glycolysis predominates:

■ during the first 2 minutes of exercise (excluding the first few seconds during which energy demands are met by direct ATP breakdown)

■ in the middle of any activity—even prolonged ones— where an increase in intensity raises the energy requirements above that which can be met aerobically

Running an 800 meter, doing 12 reps of Bench Press, and kicking to pass a competitor during a 10K are all primarily powered by anaerobic glycolysis. It supports short-term, high-intensity exercise.

The *Short-Term* Energy Source

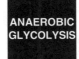

Provides energy for...

■ the first 2 minutes of exercise

■ increases in intensity to above the maximum aerobic level

LOW INTENSITY, LONG DURATION

Finally, aerobic processes, including aerobic glycolysis, meet our *long-term* energy requirements. Aerobic glycolysis is often called the *long-term* **energy source**. As long as you can meet most of an activity's energy demands aerobically, you can keep going for days (theoretically, at least). You have plenty of raw fuel in the form of available carbohydrate, protein, and fat, and none of the factors that can interfere with prolonged energy production (which we'll consider in a moment) enter into the picture.

Running a marathon, pedaling 15 to 90 minutes on the exercise bike and doing aerobic dance are all powered primarily by aerobic energy production.

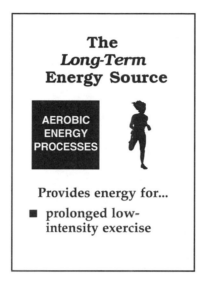

The Long-Term Energy Source

AEROBIC ENERGY PROCESSES

Provides energy for...
■ prolonged low-intensity exercise

As we said at the beginning of this chapter, all three forms of energy production contribute during most activities. But there is a basic progression from one form to the next.

During a strictly low-intensity activity such as jogging, energy production progresses from a mainly aerobic resting state to mainly direct ATP breakdown (as exercise begins), to being mainly anaerobic (as direct ATP breakdown slows), and finally, back to being mainly aerobic—although at a much higher level than at rest (as the cardiovascular system gets up to speed) (Fig. 4).

MEMBERS OF THE SAME TEAM

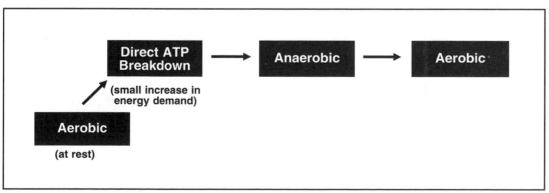

Fig. 4 — Energy Production During a Low- to Moderate-Intensity Activity

For a strictly high-intensity activity such as sprinting, energy production once again moves from a mainly aerobic resting state to mainly ATP breakdown (as exercise begins). From there, it may become mainly anaerobic—but, usually, that's as far as it goes. High-intensity activities just require too much energy (or require it too quickly) for aerobic processes to re-enter the picture (Fig. 5).

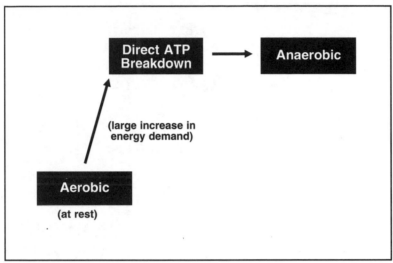

Fig. 5 — Energy Production During a High-Intensity Activity

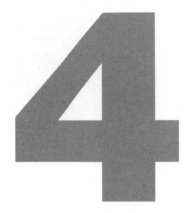

THE LACTATE THRESHOLD & VO$_2$ MAX, PART 1

When we talk about the changing balance among the types of energy production during exercise, what we're really talking about is limits—limits on anaeraobic processes, limits on aerobic processes. To round off our look at the basic forms of energy production, let's explore the far wall of each.

ANAEROBIC PROCESSES

Lactic Acid & the Lactate Threshold

Although anaerobic glycolysis does a great job supplying most of the energy for brief bursts of maximum effort, it can't sustain prolonged exercise. That's because, in addition to producing ATP, anaerobic glycolysis also produces **lactic acid**, or **lactate**, the substance that makes your legs burn at the end of a sprint. In the presence of too much lactate, energy production stops. The higher the intensity of the exercise, the faster you reach that point of no return.

Surprisingly, your body can get rid of, or **clear**, a lot of lactate by using it as a *fuel* for certain energy production processes. This is called **oxidizing** the lactate. You can get rid of even more by **buffering**. Buffering involves converting an acidic substance into something that isn't so acidic. Two compounds in the blood—**hemoglobin** (the same stuff that carries oxygen) and **bicarbonate**—are the primary buffers for lactic acid. Above a certain activity intensity level, though, the amount of lactate produced exceeds your body's ability to use or buffer it, so it accumulates, ultimately bringing energy production to a grinding halt.

That point—the point at which production exceeds removal and lactate begins to accumulate—is our infamous **lactate threshold**.* Much more on the lactate threshold in a moment.

AEROBIC PROCESSES

Steady Rate

We've said several times that when you start to exercise, your cardiovascular system takes a moment to ramp up.

In fact, over the first few minutes, oxygen consumption rises rapidly. But if the energy demands of your activity can be met aerobically, oxygen consumption quickly reaches a plateau and remains unchanged until you stop exercising or alter your pace. This plateau is called the **steady rate**. It reflects an equilibrium between the energy demands of the working muscles and the rate of aerobic ATP production. At a steady rate, little, if any, lactic acid accumulates—not because your muscles don't produce any, but because your body removes or uses the lactate as fast as it's produced.

Everyone has a **range** of potential steady rates. The breadth of that range depends on your fitness level. The diehard couch potato has a *narrow* range of steady-rate activity levels (from say, sitting in a chair to going for a leisurely walk). But the seasoned marathoner has a *wide* range—up to and including running 5-minute miles through an entire 26-mile race!

VO₂ Max

Higher steady states represent greater levels of oxygen consumption. Which brings us back to the issue of limits—just how high can you go? Research suggests the answer.

In one study, test subjects ran on a treadmill at various inclines. For the first few minutes, the treadmill was level. For the next few, it was inclined. For the next few, it was inclined further, and so on. Each subject was allowed to pick a pace appropriate to his or her condition, but the researchers made

---

*In academic circles, the lactate threshold is now referred to as *OBLA* (Onset of Blood Lactate Accumulation). We've chosen to use the more familiar *lactate threshold* because it is still the preferred term in the athletic community.

sure that the subject ran at that pace on all inclines. So, the higher the incline, the greater the demand on the subject's aerobic capacity.

Results showed that each subject's oxygen consumption rose about the same amount for each of the first three increases. That's what you would expect: greater oxygen demand, greater oxygen consumption. But for the fourth, it rose less. And for the fifth, it didn't rise at all—even though each subject continued at the same pace, and thus *had* to have been meeting the increased energy demand required by the greater inclines *somehow*.

Given that there were no further increases in oxygen consumption, clearly they weren't meeting the increased demand aerobically. This strongly suggests there *is* an upper limit on an individual's aerobic capacity. That limit—marked by the point at which oxygen consumption levels off and doesn't rise even if you increase the workload—is your **VO2 max**. Above the level represented by your VO2 max, any additional energy demands must be met anaerobically.

By the Numbers

To go much further, we need to talk numbers. Specifically, we need to put values on—and compare—*actual* VO2 maxes. So let's take a moment to get comfortable with how a VO2 max is expressed.

Your VO2 max describes the largest quantity of oxygen you can consume and use aerobically. To make that a meaningful quantity, you have to talk in terms of time—oxygen consumption *over a second, a minute, an hour,* or whatever. And you have to adjust for differences in bodyweight—oxygen consumption *per pound* or *per kilogram*. By convention, we specify VO2 max as oxygen consumption per minute and adjust for bodyweight in kilograms. That makes the actual units of VO2 max...

milliliters **of oxygen per** *kilogram* **of bodyweight per** *minute*

or

mls/kg/min

Don't worry if you don't have a sense of how much oxygen a milliliter per kilogram per minute represents. That's not important. What *is* important is understanding that:

■ Oxygen consumption, expressed in *mls/kg/min*, is a measure of how much oxygen you are using aerobically each minute, adjusted for how much you weigh

...and...

■ If you have a higher VO$_2$ max, you have a greater potential capacity to use oxygen aerobically than someone with a lower VO$_2$ max

❖

With all we just said, it would seem that your VO$_2$ max should give you a good idea how well you can perform aerobically. But it doesn't. Turns out that there's a big difference between your aerobic *capacity*, as reflected by VO$_2$ max, and your aerobic *performance ability*. In the next chapter, we'll see why.

❖　　❖　　❖

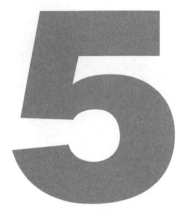

THE LACTATE THRESHOLD & VO2 MAX, PART 2

Most articles on aerobic training reflect the general acceptance of VO_2 max as the best measure of your aerobic capacity. Many even include charts showing the VO_2 "maxes" of various kinds of athletes and seem to suggest that you should work your own VO_2 max up to the appropriate level for your sport.

There are two problems with this. First, the absolute limits on VO_2 max seem to be genetically determined, so you may not be *able* to work up to some world-class athlete's VO_2 max. Second—and more important—contrary to popular belief, VO_2 max alone doesn't determine your ability to *perform* aerobically! It is a good *indicator* of overall health and fitness, but doesn't necessarily reflect total aerobic fitness or performance capacity.

Here's why.

We just described a study in which subjects ran on a treadmill at progressively higher inclines. Remember that each subject eventually reached a point at which oxygen consumption leveled off even though the workload continued to increase. This leveling off, we said, reflected each subject's VO_2 max.

Well, what we didn't say was that most of these people were *hurting* at that point. All were experiencing major lactate accumulation and serious muscle pain. If the researchers hadn't been there egging the subjects on, and if the subjects hadn't agreed in advance to keep going even if they became uncomfortable, these folks would have stopped running well before the fifth incline.

In other words: *For most people, VO$_2$ max is way above the highest activity level at which they can achieve a steady rate and continue to perform aerobically.* That level—their maximum aerobic *performance* level—depends on the way VO$_2$ max interacts with (you guessed it) the lactate threshold.

Current research shows we produce lactate all the time. Even during a slow jog, some anaerobic metabolism occurs. However, because of the activity's low ongoing energy demands, you stay below your lactate threshold and no lactic acid accumulates.

If you increase the pace, though, anaerobic energy production delivers a progressively greater proportion of energy. Your muscles produce more lactic acid. Step up the pace still further and at some point you cross over your lactate threshold—*even though you may be nowhere close to your VO$_2$ max.* Lactate accumulates; you're forced to stop your run.

What's interesting here is that we've identified a limit on aerobic activity that has nothing to do with the availablity of oxygen or your VO$_2$ max. It's lactate accumulation—not limited oxygen—that brings you to a screeching halt! That single fact provides the basis for the **Max O$_2$** way of looking at aerobic training.

Let's put some numbers on the relationship between VO$_2$ max and the lactate threshold.

The average sedentary individual has a VO$_2$ max anywhere from 20 to 40 mls/kg/min and a lactate threshold at about 50% of their VO$_2$ max.

If you have a VO$_2$ max of 40 mls/kg/min and an average lactate threshold of 50%, you'll do fine with activities requiring no more than about 20 mls/kg/min. When walking below the 20 mls/kg/min level, you'll be able to go on for a long time, cover great distances, and carry on a full-fledged conversation.

However, if you increase your pace beyond the 20 mls/kg/min level, you'll reach your lactate threshold and lactic acid will begin to accumulate. You'll get overheated, experience local muscle pain, and have a hard time carrying on a

HOW THE LACTATE THRESHOLD AND VO$_2$ MAX ARE RELATED

conversation. Eventually, either as a result of physiological fatigue or psychological discomfort, you'll stop.

Now, assume you do some systematic aerobic training and increase your lactate threshold to 75% of your VO_2 max. Now you'll do fine with activities requiring up to 75% of 40 mls/kg/min, or 30 mls/kg/min.

Ten mls/kg/min may not sound like much improvement, but it makes a *big* difference in raising your top steady rate. Where you were walking, now you can *run*—at about double your previous pace. And you've achieved that improvement with no change in your VO_2 max!

In fact, the lactate threshold is so significant in determining performance, it's possible for someone with a *lower* VO_2 max to have a *greater* aerobic performance capacity.

Take two individuals, Jim and Joe. Say Jim has a VO_2 max of 87 mls/kg/min and Joe has one of 80 mls/kg/min. Also, say Jim has a lacate threshold at 75%; Joe, at 85%. That means Jim has a performance capacity of 65 mls/kg/min, while Joe, with the lower VO_2 max, winds up with the *higher* performance capacity of 68 mls/kg/min.

As in our first example, it's hard to believe that a difference of 3 mls/kg/min could matter much. But when you calculate running speed based on these numbers, you find it translates into about a half mile per hour! In a marathon, a half mile per hour is a substantial difference. Joe may actually finish a good 5 to 6 blocks ahead of Jim, even though Jim has the higher VO_2 max.

Elite level athletes—marathon runners, cross-country skiers and cyclists—often have lactate thresholds at 80%, even 90%, of their VO_2 max. And it's these stratospheric lactate thresholds—combined with a very high VO_2 max as well—that allow them to perform at such high levels.

HOW MUCH IMPROVEMENT CAN YOU EXPECT?

Just how fast can you raise your VO_2 max and lactate threshold—and how much can you improve them? Obviously that's going to depend on how effectively you train. For the sake of argument, let's assume you use the **Max O_2** approach for maximum improvement on all counts.

How fast, first. Statistically, you can expect to reach your genetically determined VO_2 max within your first year of optimum training. Not everyone does, but most people do. Your lactate threshold, on the other hand, can continue to rise for several years. In fact, it will fluctuate, rising during periods of intense training, then falling back during less intense periods. If there is a level at which it tops out, it's probably quite high—above 90% of VO$_2$ max.

AVERAGE MAXIMAL OXYGEN UPTAKES (VO$_2$ MAX*) OF TEAM NATIONAL ATHLETES

EVENT	MEN	WOMEN
Cross-Country Skiing	82	63
Running 3000 meters (appr. 2 mi.)	79	—
Speed Skating	78	54
Orienteering	77	59
Running 800-1500 meters	75	—
Bicycling	74	—
Biathlon	73	—
Walking	71	—
Canoeing	70	—
Downhill Skiing	68	51
Running 400 meters	67	56
Swimming	66	57
Ski Jumping	62	—
Rowing	62	—
Gymnastics	60	—
Table Tennis	58	44
Fencing	58	43
Wrestling	56	—
Weight Lifting	55	—
Archery	—	40
Untrained	43	39

*mls/kg/min

Maximal Oxygen Uptake in Athletes
B. Saltin & P. Astrand
Journal of Applied Physiology
V 23 # 3: 353-358, Sept. 1967

The currently accepted top for improvement in VO$_2$ max is somewhere between 20% and 40%. Some individuals make 50% to 100% improvements, but those folks are rare, indeed! That means that if you're an average individual with a VO$_2$ max of 40 mls/kg/min, you can reasonably expect to increase it to 48 to 56 mls/kg/min. See the chart above to get a sense of where that would put your aerobic capacity relative to world-class aerobic athletes.

And lactate threshold? Since this is always measured in terms of a percentage of VO$_2$ max and, at least during the first year, your VO$_2$ max is changing, as well, it's difficult to assign an exact number here. We can say that for some of the factors that contribute to a higher threshold (mitochondrial density and volume, capillary density and volume, and aerobic enzyme factors in the individual muscle fibers), it's not unusual to see a two- to three-fold increase.

...all of which is to say that, by following the **Max O$_2$** approach to training and addressing both VO$_2$ max *and* lactate threshold, you can make a whopping big difference in your aerobic capacity!

❖　　❖　　❖

FIBER TYPE & EXERCISE

We have one more piece of the puzzle to drop into place. In a way, it's the most important piece, because it's the one that determines the basic guidelines for optimum aerobic training. It explains why bodybuilders *must* do long, slow aerobic sessions but should *never* do high-intensity, prolonged aerobic work. It explains why endurance athletes and people trying to lose weight *can't* just spend hours on the exercise bike. And it explains why some people are just better at aerobic exercise than others.

It's a matter of muscle anatomy....

MUSCLE STRUCTURE

Muscles vary greatly in size and shape, from the massive ones controlling locomotion (gluteis, hamstrings, quadriceps, and others) to the minuscule ones of the inner ear. But at a microscopic level, all are very similar in form and function.

Muscles are organized structurally in 6 levels (see Fig. 6, on the next page). At the highest level is the whole muscle; at the lowest, the thick and thin filaments of contractile and regulatory proteins—actin, myosin, tropomyosin, troponin, and others—that form the basis for muscle contraction. In between (at level 3) lies probably the most familiar of muscle's structural elements: the muscle *fiber*.

LEVELS OF MUSCLE ORGANIZATION

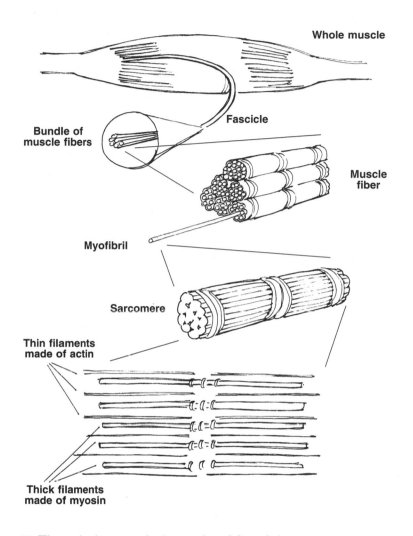

Whole muscle

Fascicle

Bundle of muscle fibers

Muscle fiber

Myofibril

Sarcomere

Thin filaments made of actin

Thick filaments made of myosin

- ◼ The whole muscle is made of **fascicles**
- ◼ Each fascicle is made of **muscle fibers**
- ◼ Each muscle fiber is made of **myofibrils**
- ◼ Each myofibril is made of **sarcomeres** laid end-to-end
- ◼ Each sarcomere is made of overlapping **thick** and **thin filaments**
- ◼ The thick and thin filaments are made of the proteins **myosin** and **actin**

Fig. 6 — Muscles are organized in 6 levels.

MUSCLE FIBER TYPES

Not all muscle fibers are created equal. In humans, there are three main types:

- Type 1
- Type 2A
- Type 2B

Each has its own characteristics.

Type 1 fibers are slow to contract but slow to fatigue. Type 2A are fast to contract and intermediate to fatigue. Type 2B are fast to contract and fast to fatigue.

One reason the Type 1 fibers are slow to fatigue is that they contain more **mitochondria**. Mitochondria are the "factories" within muscle cells that produce energy aerobically from glucose. Having more mitochondria, they are able to produce more energy. This makes them tire less quickly. Type 1 fibers are also smaller in diameter than Type 2A and 2B fibers and have greater capillary blood flow around them. These factors improve oxygen delivery and waste-product removal from the fibers, also making them tire less quickly.

Recruitment

When a muscle begins to contract, the fibers don't all contract at once. Mostly Type 1 fibers fire first, then Type 2A, then 2B. This sequence of fiber **recruitment** allows very delicate and finely tuned muscle responses to brain commands. But it also makes Type 2B fibers difficult to train—because most of the Type 1 and 2A fibers have to be working before many of the 2B fibers participate. The importance of that fact will be obvious in a moment.

RESPONSE TO AEROBIC EXERCISE

The way all muscle fibers adapt to exercise depends on the way you work out. When you do endurance work, the main response is *increased capacity for energy production*.

The increase is due to the development of:

- more energy-producing enzymes in the mitochondria
- more mitochondria
- bigger mitochondria

Interestingly enough, if the intensity of that exercise is less than about 50% of VO_2 max, only Type 1 (also known as **slow-twitch**) fibers are affected. Type 2A and 2B fibers are not. To target Type 2 (also known as **fast-twitch**) fibers, *you must exercise close to maximum intensity.* This makes sense in light of the recruitment pattern mentioned a moment ago: Remember, as exercise intensity increases, the Type 1, then 2A, then 2B fibers are sequentially activated. Once the 2As kick in, you are operating at, or slightly below, your lactate threshold.

Targeting Different Fiber Types

While all muscle fibers respond to endurance exercise by increasing their capacity for energy production, they respond to resistance exercise (weight lifting, working with rubber straps, etc.) by getting bigger. Again, there's a threshold for Type 2 involvement—at about 70% of your one-rep max for the muscles involved.

Muscle hypertrophy (increased size) is mostly the result of more protein being deposited in level 4 of your muscle structure, the myofibrils, as well as more water and glycogen being stored there. Resistance training builds up the myofibrils in both fast- and slow-twitch fibers, but appears to affect fast-twitch fibers more.*

In contrast to the response to endurance exercise, resistance exercise causes a *decrease* in mitochondrial volume and the enzymes of energy production. These changes can reduce endurance in athletes who do nothing but lift weights.

RESPONSE TO RESISTANCE EXERCISE

Can training change the relative balance of fast-twitch to slow-twitch fibers in a muscle? In general, no—a muscle's fiber composition is mostly determined by your genes. So, sprinters (who have a high percentage of fast-twitch fibers in their muscles) and marathoners (who have a high percent-

CAN FIBER TYPE BE CHANGED?

*Long-term resistance training may increase overall muscle size not only by increasing fiber size (fiber *hypertrophy*) but also by increasing fiber number (fiber *hyperplasia*). However, the current belief is that hyperplasia—if it occurs at all—is a relatively minor contributor; most of the increase in size seems to come from fiber hypertrophy.

age of slow-twitch fibers) most likely have the fiber compositions they do mainly because they are genetically programmed to. In other words, successful sprinters are successful because they are born with a high percentage of fast-twitch fibers, not because they developed them with training.

However, although you probably can't turn a slow-twitch fiber into a fast-twitch one (or vice versa),* **you can make one fiber type take on *characteristics* of the other under certain circumstances.** As we'll see below, this has *profound* implications for your training.

OVERTRAINING

One final point before we look at the significance of fiber type in optimizing aerobic programs.

All the adaptations we just mentioned—increases in contractile protein in response to resistance exercise, increases in capillarization and mitochondrial density in response to endurance exercise, and so on—can be inhibited by overzealous conditioning. Adaptation is part of recovery; it happens while you *rest*. If you consistently allow insufficient recovery time between training sessions, you can retard your progress or even lose ground. This is called **overtraining** and is probably the number-one roadblock to athletic success.

Although you can overtrain by overdoing exercise at any duration or intensity, *it's most likely to occur after repeated, prolonged, high-intensity sessions.*

There's also a way you can overtrain in the short term. High-intensity training depletes both muscle and liver glycogen. Inadequate recovery time can interfere with glycogen replenishment, leading to decreased energy during a subsequent training session. This effect is especially pronounced if you're eating the kind of low-calorie, low-carbohydrate diet preferred by pre-contest bodybuilders and people trying to lose weight.

Those facts, as well, have profound implications with regards to muscle fibers and your training.

---

*Some recent evidence suggests that many years of systematic training may in fact cause a *limited* amount of fiber conversion; this finding is not considered conclusive.

Hidden in the discussion above are the facts that determine how to match aerobics training to your goal. Let's see if we can uncover them now.

We said that all muscle fibers—fast twitch and slow—may participate during all kinds of activities, but that the fast-twitch fibers only participate if an activity demands more than about 50% of VO_2 max (or 70% of one-rep max if we're talking about resistance exercise). We also said that too much high-intensity work increases risk of overtraining.

So consider this scenario:

You're a bodybuilder and you've been killing yourself to pile on the mass for an upcoming physique contest. In fact, you've been concentrating so hard on size that you've waited too long to start your pre-contest-lose-bodyfat-aerobic regimen. To make up for lost time, you ride the bike or jog at a higher intensity than you normally would, figuring that will take off the fat faster.

In fact, you push yourself so hard that you spend the better part of 8 weeks doing continuous aerobic work well above the 50% threshold. The high-intensity training brings the fast-twitch fibers into play. *Now they're contributing during your aerobic work as well as your resistance training.* And zap! You begin to lose leg mass as the 2As and 2Bs become both glycogen-depleted and overtrained from a schedule allowing inadequate time for recovery. **In general, prolonged high-intensity aerobic work is likely to decrease the size of the involved muscles. That's why bodybuilders should stear clear of high-intensity aerobic sessions.**

The facts fit together a bit differently for aerobic athletes.

Recall that short-duration, high-intensity training—sprinting, lifting weights, and the like—exaggerates the characteristics of fast-twitch fibers: it causes myofibril volume to go *up* and the size and number of mitochondria to go *down*. In effect, short-duration, high-intensity training causes all muscle fibers to become more "fast-twitch-like." They get *better* at faster, high-intensity contractions and *worse* at prolonged aerobic work.

So consider a second scenario.

You're an aerobic athlete who's become bored with all the prolonged, low-intensity work. You figure you'll take a season off to hit the gym—to do heavy squats, leg extensions, and leg curls (and no long, steady distance)—in the hopes that the increased leg strength will improve your endurance. In fact, you

WHY FIBER TYPE MATTERS

so enjoy lifting that 12 to 18 months go by before you get back on the track. And once again, zap! Although the increased leg strength gives you the *potential* to be faster and have greater local muscular endurance, you find that, in fact, you have *less* local endurance. That's because, due to the conversion effect we've been talking about, the 2A and 2B fibers (and to some extent, the Type 1s) have become better suited to resistance exercise than endurance exercise (not to mention that your VO$_2$ max has taken a nose dive after a year and a half of no long, steady distance training!).

The bottom line: The right kind of training can enhance your performance; the wrong kind can undermine your athletic success. Your progress depends on your making the right choices in setting up your aerobic program.

❖

With fiber conversion covered, the stage is set to lay out the guidelines for optimum aerobic training. That's what we're going to do in the next chapter, after tying fiber conversion in with all the topics covered so far—the cardiovascular system, energy processes by fuel involved, energy processes by type, VO$_2$ max, and the lactate threshold.

❖   ❖   ❖

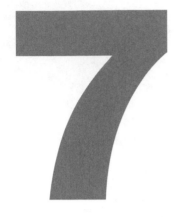

SOME ASSEMBLY REQUIRED

It's time for that last page of the mystery we referred to in Chapter 1. Let's see how all the puzzle pieces interlock to form the basis for **Max O₂** aerobics work. First we'll list the pieces, then assemble them. The list below will also serve as a review of the 11 key points covered so far.

THE PIECES

The Cardiovascular System

❶ **The cardiovascular system** is responsible for the uptake and delivery of oxygen to the muscles for use in aerobic energy production. It is also responsible for the removal of certain energy-production waste products, most notably carbon dioxide and water.

ATP

❷ All energy for physiological processes comes from "burning" **ATP**. You have about 3 ounces of ATP available for immediate use. After that gets used up, more ATP must be synthesized via various processes using carbohydrate, fat, or protein as "fuels."

❸ There are basically three kinds of energy production processes: **non-aerobic** (the direct use of ATP), **anaerobic** (making new ATP without oxygen), and **aerobic** (making new ATP with oxygen).

Energy Production

❹ Although anaerobic processes can produce ATP quickly, they also produce **lactic acid**, or **lactate**. Above a certain activity intensity level, you make more lactic acid than you can use or remove, so it begins to accumulate. Ultimately, this can bring activity to a halt. The activity intensity level at which lactic acid starts to accumulate is called your **lactate threshold**.

Lactate Threshold

❺ For a range of prolonged, low-intensity activities, you can meet most of the ATP demands aerobically. If you start up any of those activities and keep at it at a consistent pace, your oxgyen consumption (reflecting the oxygen demand) rises to a particular level and then basically stays there. This is called achieving a **steady rate**.

Steady Rate

❻ There is a ceiling on your aerobic energy production reflected by your **VO$_2$ max**. Below your VO$_2$ max, oxgyen consumption *increases* if you work harder. Above VO$_2$ max, oxygen consumption *remains the same* if you work harder because aerobic energy production has maxed out. Once you're operating above your VO$_2$ max, any additional energy demands must be met anaerobically.

VO$_2$ Max

❼ There is a difference between your **aerobic capacity**, as measured in a lab, and your **aerobic performance ability**, as experienced when you're actually trying to *do* something aerobic—such as run a 10K or cycle 100 miles. Your laboratory aerobic capacity is determined by your VO$_2$ max. Your practical aerobic performance ability is determined by the combination of your VO$_2$ max and your lactate threshold. It's (usually) much lower than your VO$_2$ max.

Aerobic Capacity vs.
Aerobic Performance Ability

❽ Muscle basically consists of three kinds of fibers: **Type 1**, **Type 2A** and **Type 2B**. The Type 1s, also known as *slow-twitch* fibers, are best suited to prolonged, low-intensity activity. They:

Muscle Fiber Type and Exercise

- are smaller
- produce less force
- have a more extensive blood supply

■ contain more mitochondria

The Type 2As and 2Bs, also known as *fast-twitch* fibers, are better suited to short-term, high-intensity activity. They:

■ are larger
■ produce more force
■ contain more contractile protein
■ have a less extensive blood supply and fewer mito-chondria
■ produce significantly more lactate than the Type 1s

Although both the Type 2A and 2B fibers share fast-twitch characteristics, the 2As are "less fast-twitch-like" than the 2Bs.

Recruitment

❾ As activity intensity rises, your nervous system **recruits** the Type 1 fibers first, then the Type 2As, then the 2Bs.

Fiber "Pseudo-Conversion"

❿ It's probably not possible to actually turn a Type 1 fiber into a Type 2 fiber (or vice versa), but prolonged high-intensity aerobic work *can* make Type 2 fibers more Type-1-like. Similarly, consistent short-duration, high-intensity anaerobic work can make the Type 1 fibers more Type-2-like.

Overtraining

⓫ Excessive training plus inadequate recovery time can lead to a condition known as **overtraining**, in which the body's ability to adapt to the stress of exercise is impaired. It can also result in glycogen depletion that interferes with your ability to train intensely.

ASSEMBLY IN PROGRESS

As you've undoubtedly picked up by now, all 11 factors listed above are tightly interrelated. The key element that ties them all together is *fiber type*. Here's how.

The Type 1 Intensity Range

Each of us has a range of low-intensity activities for which we can produce most of the required ATP aerobically. Sure, even within this range, you generate some of the energy anaerobically, but aerobic energy production predominates.

Activities fall within this range if, at your fitness level, the **Type 1 fibers** (the slow, highly vascular, relatively smaller fibers—the ones that get recruited first) can do most of the work. Since the Type 1 fibers don't produce much lactic acid—and since your body can easily use or buffer what little is generated—exercise within this range doesn't result in a rise in blood lactate. In other words, it takes place **well below lactate threshold**.

Everyone **can achieve a steady rate** within this range.*

The Type 2A Intensity Range

As intensity rises, though, the picture changes. At some intermediate level, the load is too great for the Type 1s to handle, so the Type 2As get into the act. (This corresponds to the point at which, if you were running, you would begin having trouble carrying on a normal conversation.)

Remember that the Type 2s are better suited to anaerobic energy production than the Type 1s. In producing more energy anaerobically, the Type 2As also produce more lactic acid. In fact, they produce enough that some begins to accumulate—which means that once the Type 2As start contributing, you're operating at, or just below, your lactate threshold.

For a certain range of intensities starting here and going up a ways, you can still use or buffer enough of the lactic acid so that blood lactate doesn't rise out of control. Instead, it plateaus. You experience some localized muscle fatigue, an elevated breathing rate, and other effects consistent with being at or just below the lacate threshold.

Almost everyone **can achieve a steady rate** within this range.**

The Type 2B Intensity Range

Pump up the intensity still further, and the balance tips strongly in favor of anaerobic energy production. Here, both the 2As *and* 2Bs get recruited. And while the 2Bs are well-equipped to meet very high energy demands via anaerobic glycolysis, they generate *a lot* of lactate.

*For those who like numbers, exercise in this domain is usually associated with lactate concentrations of 1 to 2 millimolar.

**Exercise within the 2A domain is usually associated with lactate concentrations up to 4 millimolar.

Once the 2B fibers get involved, you're operating well above your lactate threshold. At this level, the amount of lactate your muscles produce can quickly overwhelm your body's clearing ability. So, in short order, you either have to slow down or stop completely (depending on how much pain you can stand).

No one can achieve a steady rate operating this far above the lactate threshold. But advanced aerobic athletes can tolerate the pain associated with working with some lactic acid present, so they can still perform for a limited time in this range.*

ASSEMBLED AND READY TO ROLL

One more time in many fewer words...

- As long as the Type 1 fibers can do most of the work, energy production remains largely aerobic. You operate below your lactate threshold. Blood lactate level doesn't rise.

- As intensity increases, eventually the Type 2As are forced to kick in, so more energy is produced anaerobically. There is *some* rise in blood lactate. Rather than rising out of control, though, your blood lactate level plateaus. You are operating at, or just below, your lactate threshold.

- If intensity rises still further and the 2Bs have to get into the act, energy production becomes largely anaerobic. All three fiber types contribute, but the 2As and 2Bs do most of the work. Your blood lactate level rises dramatically and steadily until you can't continue. You are operating well above your lactate threshold.

Theory Meets Practice

So, what does *any* of this have to do with training?

Most sports require performance in all three ranges associated with the three fiber types. And given that your body responds very specifically to the kind of exercise you do, you can't expect to improve your performance significantly in all

---

*Exercise within the 2B domain is usually associated with lactate concentrations above 4 millimolar. Recreational athletes can tolerate up to about 15 millimolar; world-class athletes can tolerate up to 25 to 30 millimolar.

three ranges using just one kind of exercise. In fact, long, steady distance, which is mostly a Type 1 activity, does just what you might expect: Assuming you're moderately fit, it improves your ability to perform in the Type 1 range. It does *not* significantly improve your ability to perform at or above your lactate threshold.*

To accomplish that goal, you need to do exercises that specifically target the fiber type and energy production mechanisms involved at or above your lactate threshold—or you'll never achieve your full aerobic potential.

One more fish to throw in the kettle. Remember *fiber conversion*—the effect of prolonged, high-intensity aerobic work making Type 2 fibers more Type-1-like, and short-duration, high-intensity anaerobic work making Type 1 fibers more Type-2-like (point #10 on our summary list three pages back)?

Well, the fact of fiber conversion, along with overtraining, puts some definite limits on how you apply our three-pronged approach to aerobic work. And that brings us to the true bottom line. The complete, everything-included (even the Ginsu knives), specific aerobic training guidelines that underlie the **Max O2** approach—applied to the four basic goals defined in the introduction (bodybuilding, losing weight, getting fit, and preparing for an endurance event such as a marathon)—are as follows:

Bodybuilding

If you're a bodybuilder, you want to drop bodyfat to almost subhuman levels, while building—or at least maintaining—muscle mass. Almost all forms of aerobic training will help you drop bodyfat.** But to limit muscle-size loss due to glycogen depletion and the overtraining of the fast-twitch fibers, you want to keep the Type 2A and 2B fibers out of the act—in other words, you want to do your aerobic work well below your lactate threshold.

---

*Long, steady distance will improve both VO2 max *and* lactate threshold in extremely unfit individuals.

**Swimming may be the one exception. Some research shows less bodyfat lost from burning a particular number of calories swimming than from burning that same number of calories doing other aerobic exercises. More on this later in the *Training* Section.

Losing Weight

If you're significantly overweight, you probably want to drop the extra pounds as fast as possible. Ultimately, that means you want to be able to exercise aerobically for long periods at a high intensity—*not a low one*—because the pounds will come off faster if you're burning more calories during each workout.

Chances are, though, that you're not in such great shape to begin with. In fact, you may not even be able to do low-intensity work for more than a few minutes at a time. Developing the ability to do the kind of prolonged sessions necessary for weight loss will require a special approach we'll discuss in the next section.

Ultimately, though, you want to *encourage* the metabolic changeover that makes fast-twitch fibers more slow-twitch-like so you can do prolonged aerobic work at a high intensity. Again, this calls for training in at least the Type 1 and Type 2A ranges. But unlike the endurance athlete, you don't need to develop world-class aerobic performance capacity or a finishing kick, so you can stay away from Type 2B work.*

Improving Fitness

If you're just trying to get fit, you want to strike a balance between increasing your aerobic performance capacity and building some muscle mass to promote improved physical capabilities and appearance. This will involve mostly Type 1, low-intensity work, with a little lactate-threshold training thrown in for good measure (but not enough to cause major metabolic conversion of your 2A and 2B fibers).

Preparing for an Endurance Event

And finally, if you're an endurance athlete, you want to build the highest possible aerobic performance capacity. That requires maximizing the aerobic capabilities of *both* your slow-twitch *and* fast-twitch fibers. In other words, you want to *encourage* the metabolic changeover that makes fast-twitch fibers more slow-twitch-like. Improving the aerobic capabilities of both fast- and slow-twitch fibers involves training in all three intensity ranges. The Type 1 and Type 2A work raises the highest steady rate you can sustain, allowing you to run your entire event at a faster pace without exceeding your

---

*There is a high-intensity training method involving the 2Bs that can increase your rate of weight loss dramatically. We'll cover it in the *Training* Section.

lactate threshold. And the Type 2B work builds you a mighty kick to put you first at the finish line.

❖

That's it! Those are the basic **Max O₂** guidelines. In the up-coming *Training* section, we will explore how to use them to optimize your aerobic workout program.

❖   ❖   ❖

PART TWO

Training

IDENTIFYING YOUR RISK FACTORS

All forms of physical conditioning carry a certain risk. But because aerobic training involves raising your heart rate—often substantially—for long periods, it has the potential to cause more serious physical harm than many other forms of training. It should therefore be approached with caution and an awareness of any factors that might increase that risk. As a first step toward using the **Max O₂** program, evaluate your risk by following the directions below and referring to the information and recommendations supplied by the *American College of Sports Medicine (A.C.S.M.)*.

❶ Consult the list of *risk factors* and the list of *symptoms* on the next page.

❷ Use the information from those lists and the Risk Classification Guidelines on page 56 to determine your risk classification.

❸ Check whether your risk classification indicates you should have a medical exam and exercise stress test before beginning an aerobic program (and whether a physician should be present during such a test) by looking up your risk classification in the chart also on page 56.

As a cross-check, you should answer the questionnaire in the box on page 57, too.

If you identify any risk factors for yourself, consult with your physician before beginning aerobic training. Likewise, if you have any doubt about your present condition, medical history, or risk classification, see your physician.

A.C.S.M. MAJOR RISK FACTORS

■ Diagnosed hypertension or systolic blood pressure at or above 160 mmHg, or a diastolic blood pressure at or above 90 mmHg

■ Serum cholesterol at or greater than 240 mg/dl

■ Smoking

■ Diabetes Mellitus (Persons with insulin-dependent diabetes mellitus {IDDM} who are over the age of 30, or have had IDDM for more than 15 years, and persons with non-insulin dependent diabetes mellitus who are over 35 years of age should be classified as patients with disease and treated according to the *With Disease* guidelines in the chart on page 56.)

■ Family history of coronary disease or other artherosclerotic disease in parents or siblings prior to age 55

A.C.S.M. SYMPTOMS OR SIGNS SUGGESTIVE OF DISEASE

■ Pain or discomfort in the chest or surrounding areas that appears to be ischemic in nature

■ Unaccustomed shortness of breath or shortness of breath on mild exertion

■ Dizziness or passing out

■ Difficulty breathing at night while sleeping

■ Swollen ankles

■ Palpitations or rapid heart rate

■ Limping or lameness

■ Known heart murmur

I

A.C.S.M. RISK CLASSIFICATION

Apparently Healthy

Free of symptoms; no more than one
major risk factor

AT Higher Risk

Symptoms suggestive of cardiopulmonary or
metabolic disease and/or two or more
major risk factors

With Disease

Those with known cardiopulmonary or
metabolic disease

I

AGE BREAKS Men ≤ 40 Women ≤ 50	APPARENTLY HEALTHY		HIGHER RISK		
	Younger	Older	No Symptoms	Symptoms	WITH DISEASE
Medical exam and diagnostic exercise test recommended prior to...					
Moderate Exercise	Not Necessary	Not Necessary	Not Necessary	Yes	Yes
Vigorous Exercise	Not Necessary	Yes	Yes	Yes	Yes
Physician supervision recommended during test...					
Sub-Maximal Testing	Not Necessary	Not Necessary	Not Necessary	Yes	Yes
Maximal Testing	Not Necessary	Yes	Yes	Yes	Yes

Fig. 7 — A.C.S.M. Guidelines for Exercise Testing and Participaton

I

PHYSICAL ACTIVITY READINESS QUESTIONNAIRE (PAR-Q)

For most people, physical activity should not pose any problem or hazard. The PAR-Q has been designed to identify the small number of adults for whom physical activity might be inappropriate or those who should have medical advice before proceeding with a change in activity.

- Has a doctor ever said you have heart trouble?
- Do you frequently suffer from pains in your chest?
- Do you often feel faint or have spells of severe dizziness?
- Has a doctor ever said your blood pressure was too high?
- Has a doctor ever told you you have a bone or joint problem such as arthritis that has been aggravated by exercise, or might be made worse by exercise?
- Is there a good physical reason not mentioned here why you should not start an activity program even if you wanted to?
- Are you over 65 years old and not accustomed to vigorous exercise?

If you answered *yes* to any of these questions, postpone vigorous exercise or testing until you check with our doctor.

Chisholm, D.M., Collis, M.L., Culac, L.L.,
Davenport, W., Grube, N.;
Physical Activity Readiness;
Br Col Med J; 17:375-378, 1975

❖   ❖   ❖

THE MAX O$_2$ BUILDING BLOCKS

OK. Let's get to work. We're going to cut right to the chase with an overview of the **Max O$_2$** building blocks. Then we'll go back and explore them in detail.

Regardless of your specific objective, the basic goals of **Max O$_2$** are the same—training to:

- increase your VO$_2$ max
- elevate your lactate threshold

IMPROVING VO$_2$ MAX

Recall that VO$_2$ max reflects your body's capacity to produce energy aerobically. Studies show you can increase this capacity using a broad range of training intensities, both below and above your lactate threshold. But most people find training above the lactate threshold *very* uncomfortable. Indeed, few individuals are likely to stick with any program that requires them to suffer such discomfort, day in and day out, even for brief periods.

Training below the lactate threshold, on the other hand—doing prolonged, low-intensity work—ultimately will get you the same improvement in VO$_2$ max without a lot of the pain. It just takes a little longer to get there.

So—the first building block of the **Max O₂** approach, the only one that's also part of the traditional aerobics training model, is the use of prolonged, low-intensity exercise to improve VO₂ max.

MAX O₂ BUILDING BLOCK #1

Technique: Prolonged, low-intensity exercise

Basic Goal: Improving VO₂ max

Fiber Involvement: Type 1

Effect: Increases (mainly) Type 1 fiber oxidative capacity, also cardio-pulmonary capacity, hormonal response, and capillarization; also improves thermal response, muscular endurance, and body composition

---

TRAINING TO RAISE YOUR LACTATE THRESHOLD

Lactate-threshold training requires a completely different approach. Your lactate threshold is at or above the point at which the Type 2A fibers begin to be recruited. To work the Type 2s—and raise your lactate threshold—you can't just use the traditional long, steady distance approach. You have to train at or above your lactate threshold.

Depending on your specific training goal, lactate threshold training will involve any or all of three techniques: **threshold runs**, **intervals**, and **peaking threshold runs**.

Threshold Runs

Threshold runs involve long aerobic sessions performed right at your lactate threshold. They typically last from 20 to 40 minutes. Yes, this is hard. But the purpose of threshold runs is to simulate race conditions. So unless you're training for an endurance event, you probably won't need them in your program.

MAX O₂ BUILDING BLOCK #2

Technique: Threshold Runs

Basic Goal: Raising the lactate threshold, especially for activities involving prolonged, high-intensity activity

Fiber Involvement: Type 1 and Type 2A

Effect: Improves oxidative capacity of additional Type 1 fibers not recruited during LSD training; also increases the oxidative capacity of many (and potentially all) 2A fibers

---

Intervals

Intervals are just what they sound like—alternating periods of activity and rest. For example, you might run hard for 5 minutes, then walk for 2. Then run for another 5 minutes, then walk for 2. And so on. Intervals can be used below, at, or above lactate threshold, and even above VO₂ max. Your sport or fitness goal determines the best choice of actual activity, intensity of activity, and balance between activity and rest.

MAX O₂ BUILDING BLOCK #3

Technique: Intervals

Goal: Raising the lactate threshold

Fiber Involvement: Type 2B

Effect: Improves lactate clearance and tolerance of (mainly) the Type 2B fibers; also increases the lactate buffering capacity of the blood, liver, and kidneys

---

Peaking threshold runs are even more intense. They're any *combination* of sprints plus threshold runs. For example, you might start your 20-to-40-minute threshold run, then, say every 3 minutes, sprint for 30 seconds, then "rest" by dropping back to the threshold-run pace. Or you might just do a series of intervals followed immediately by a threshold run. Once again, you probably won't need to do any peaking threshold runs unless you're training for a competitive endurance event.

Peaking Threshold Runs

MAX O₂ BUILDING BLOCK #4

Technique: Peaking Threshold Runs

Goal: Raising the lactate threshold, especially for activities involving prolonged, high-intensity activity and bursts of maximal activity

Fiber Involvement: Type 1, 2A & 2B

Effect: Realizes the benefits of both Threshold Runs and Intervals

---

Why three different ways to address lactate threshold training? Because of the specificity of response. Remember—the way you train must closely match the way you intend to perform. You can't improve your cycling ability by running, or your running ability by swimming, or, for that matter, your capacity to do bursts of high-intensity activity by doing long, steady distance.

Since most activities require a mix of energy demands, you need to use a mix of training methods to prepare for them.

Take boxing, for example. It requires...

■ Continuous low-intensity dancing around the ring. This is a Type 1 activity; to prepare, you need to do long, steady distance work.

■ Minutes at a time when an opponent is pressing you and you are doing the same dancing, but at a much

Applying the Three Methods of Lactate Threshold Training

higher intensity. This brings the 2A fibers into play. To prepare, you need to do threshold runs.

■ The basic 3-minute rounds alternating with short rests in your corner. This calls for interval training.

■ Periods where you are moving around at a fairly high intensity (2A fiber involvement) and then have to throw a flurry of punches (2B fiber involvement). To prepare, you need to do peaking threshold runs.

Many sports involve all four kinds of energy requirements. These demand training that includes the full complement of **Max O₂** building blocks. Other sports don't. They require a much simpler **Max O₂** program. The idea in all cases is to match the *type* of training to nature of the sport so you don't work any harder than necessary, and don't inadvertently shoot yourself in the foot by using the wrong conditioning techniques.

❖   ❖   ❖

10 LONG, STEADY DISTANCE: IMPROVING VO$_2$ MAX

In Chapters 10 and 11, we're going to discuss actually *doing* the four kinds of training touched on in the last chapter:

■ Prolonged, low-intensity training

■ Intervals

■ Threshold runs

■ Peaking threshold runs

These two chapters correspond to the *Exercises* section in other *Health For Life* courses. They cover performance of the building blocks out of which we will later fashion your program. In other words, here we will discuss a single instance of prolonged, low-intensity training, but not how many times a week or for how long to do it. Those issues will be addressed in the *Program* chapter.

Once again, let's start with improving VO$_2$ max. Remember that this requires prolonged, low-intensity training—also known as **long, steady distance work**, or **LSD**. Although *long, steady distance* sounds as if it refers to running, it can actually refer to doing *any* aerobic activity—cycling, swimming, jumping rope or whatever—for a long time at a low intensity.

QUANTITATIVE VS. INTUITIVE

Most aerobics programs use one of two approaches for LSD work. The **quantitative**, or by-the-numbers, approach bases your training on something objective, such as your heart rate. The **intuitive**, or seat-of-your-pants, approach relies on your subjective impressions—what it *feels* like while you're exercising: too hard, too easy, or just right.

Max O₂ combines the two techniques. You will use the quantitative approach to learn how it feels to do VO₂ max work at an appropriate intensity. Then you will use your educated intuitive sense of how much is enough to guide your training from that point forward.

We'll cover the quantitative approach first.

THE EXERCISE-HEART-RATE RANGE

If you've read anything about aerobic training, you're probably familiar with the idea of using a heart rate range to specify the appropriate intensity for an aerobic session. The most commonly used formula goes like this:

Take 220 minus your age to figure your maximum heart rate. Then multiply the result by 60% and 70% to set your exercise-heart-rate range.

For example, by this method, a 20-year-old would have a maximum heart rate of...

220 beats per minute (b.p.m) - 20 b.p.m. = 200 b.p.m.

...and an exercise range of...

200 b.p.m. × 60% = 120 b.p.m.
(on the low end)

— and —

200 b.p.m. × 70% = 140 b.p.m.
(on the high end)

This is called the **straight line** method for figuring exercise-heart-rate range.

We're going to use something similar to the straight line method for the VO₂ max part of your training, with a major twist. But first we have to correct for three major deficiencies in that method. In fact, we're going to use those deficiencies as our framework for laying out the **Max O₂** approach to LSD.

Missed It by *That* Much!

The first deficiency is that there's an error (what statisticians call a *standard deviation*) of plus or minus 10 b.p.m. in the 220-minus-your-age number. That means that if you take a group of 20-year-olds, their maximum heart rates will range from 190 to 210 b.p.m.

For reasons we won't go into here, that 20 b.p.m. spread doesn't matter when setting exercise guidelines for bodybuilders, for the very overweight or unfit, and for average individuals interested in getting into shape. But for world-class athletes, it can make a *big* difference in the effectiveness of an exercise prescription. If you're training for the Olympics or some other high-end event, we recommend having your maximum heart rate measured in an exercise physiology lab to ensure accuracy.* Then use the lab-determined number in the formulas that follow wherever they call for your maximum heart rate.

The Karvonen Method: Matching a Percentage of VO_2 Max

The second problem with the straight-line method is that it doesn't correlate well with the way the scientific community compares and recommends training intensities—in terms of percent of VO_2 max. In other words, training at 50% of your maximum heart rate à la straight-line does *not* mean that you're training at 50% of your VO_2 max. Figure 8 on the next page shows just how poorly these two stack up against one another.

With the huge body of useful recommendations on endurance training available, it would be nice if you and the recommendations were speaking the same language. And you easily can be. There's a simple way to improve the straight line calculation so that the exercise-range percentages do match up with VO_2 max percentages. It's called the **Karvonen Method**, and it's based on calculating exercise heart rates relative to your **heart rate reserve** (also known as your **working heart rate**), rather than to your maximum heart rate. It works like this:

Subtract your age from 220 to get your maximum heart rate. Now subtract your resting heart rate from your maximum heart rate to get your heart rate reserve. If you're very unfit, multiply by 40% and 50%, then add your resting heart rate back in. The two numbers you get are your low- and high-value exercise heart rates.

*Contact the exercise physiology department of your local college or university to find a lab where you can take the test.

Relationship Between
% Maximum Heart Rate,
% VO₂ Max, and % Heart Rate Reserve

% MAX HEART RATE (Straight Line)	% VO₂ MAX	% HEART RATE RESERVE (Karvonen)
65	50	50
68	55	55
72	60	60
76	65	65
79	70	70
83	75	75
87	80	80
91	85	85
94	90	90

Fig. 8 — Percent of Maximum Heart Rate does not match up well with Percent of VO₂ Max, but Percent of Heart Rate Reserve does.

Using Karvonen, an unfit 20-year-old with a resting heart rate of 70 would have a maximum heart rate of...

220 b.p.m - 20 b.p.m. = 200 b.p.m.

...a heart rate reserve of...

200 b.p.m - 70 b.p.m. = 130 b.p.m.

...and an exercise-heart-rate range of...

(130 b.p.m. × 40%) + 70 b.p.m. = 122 b.p.m.
(on the low end)

— and —

(130 b.p.m. × 50%) + 70 b.p.m. = 137 b.p.m.
(on the high end)

Because we've used the more exact Karvonen method and not straight-line, the guy in our example working within this range would actually be training at 40% to 50% of his VO$_2$ max.

One Man's Ceiling Is Another Man's Floor

And that brings us to the third—and by far most significant—deficiency in the straight-line method, one that's a problem for the Karvonen method, as well. You know those percentage ranges you're supposed to plug in—40% to 50% for the unfit individual, 50% to 60% for someone who's in shape, and so on? Well, they're all built on the fact that the *average* unfit person has a lactate threshold of 50% of VO$_2$ max.

Now, if your lactate threshold actually *is* 50% of VO$_2$ max, a range of 40% to 50% should keep you below it, promoting effective LSD training. But what if you *don't* have a lactate threshold of 50%? What if you're in terrible shape and you have a lactate threshold of 35%? Or, for that matter, what if you're genetically gifted and you have a lactate threshold of 65%?

For many people—especially the very unfit—training even at the 50% level represents working in the red zone. That's why you see folks in an aerobics class who can only exercise for a couple of minutes at a time, but who, when they check their pulses, have heart rates smack in the middle of their exercise-heart-rate ranges. The problem is simply that the heart-rate-range formulas don't take the lactate threshold into account.

What you really need is a way of measuring your lactate threshold heart rate. That number could then become the "ceiling" heart rate for your LSD work, and the "floor" heart rate for your lactate threshold training. And you could easily plug that number back into the Karvonen formula to get a heart rate 10% lower (to specify the bottom of a range for LSD work), or 10% higher (to specify the top of a range for lactate-threshold training). The resulting exercise-heart-rate ranges would reflect your actual current fitness level much more accurately than the numbers produced by either the straight-line or Karvonon methods.

That's exactly how the **Max O$_2$** approach to LSD works.

Here's an overview of the steps we're about to take. We're going to...

❶ Determine your lactate-threshold heart rate. This will be the *top* value of your exercise-heart-rate range for LSD.

❷ Plug your lactate-threshold heart rate into a modified version of the Karvonen formula to get the percentage of VO_2 max it represents.

❸ Calculate the heart rate representing 10% less than the value we got in ❷. This will be the *bottom* value of your exercise-heart-rate range for LSD.

❹ Start training!

You can determine your lactate-threshold heart rate in one of four ways. You can have a rather uncomfortable blood-analysis/treadmill test done where a researcher systematically raises the treadmill speed and draws blood at each increase, looking for an elevation in lactate (don't worry; we're not recommending this); you can take any of a number of performance-related tests, such as the *Test Conconi*; you can go out and experiment to find the fastest pace at which you can run for a maximum of 15 minutes and measure your heart rate at that pace; or you can simply use the **Talk Test**.

The Talk Test involves running, cycling, jumping rope or whatever faster and faster until you begin to have difficulty carrying on a conversation. If you take your pulse right at that moment, you get your lactate-threshold heart rate. That's all there is to it. Here's how to take the test....

❶ Pick the exercise you're going to use for your aerobic training. If possible, find yourself a partner who won't mind doing that activity with you for a few minutes.

❷ Go out and run, cycle, jump or whatever very, very slowly for at least 5 minutes to get your system up to speed. If you have a partner, carry on a conversation with them as you rev up; if not, talk to yourself *out loud* as if you were talking to someone else. (That's why we recommend the partner; you'll look a little goofy doing this alone.)

If, even at this very slow start-up speed, you can't carry on a conversation, decrease the intensity or pick a less intense

THE *MAX O₂* APPROACH TO LSD

Determining Your Lactate-Threshold Heart Rate

The Talk Test

activity. For example, drop back to walking if jogging puts you over the edge.

❸ Now, slowly increase the intensity (by walking or jogging faster) until you begin having trouble carrying on a conversation. At that point—technically known as the onset of **unstable ventilation**—take your pulse. We advise taking it at your wrist, rather than at your neck. There is a physiological reflex associated with pressure on the carotid artery than can lower your pulse and give you inaccurate results. Memorize the number you get. Then slow down until you can carry on a conversation once again.

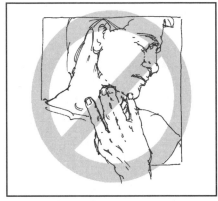

Fig. 9 — For maximum accuracy, take your pulse at your wrist, not your neck

Repeat this cycle 2 more times so that, in the end, you have 3 heart-rate numbers corresponding to the 3 times you reached the intensity at which it became difficult to carry on a conversation. Write those numbers in the box below. Add them up. And divide by 3 to get their average. That number is your heart rate at your lactate threshold.

Calculating Your Threshold Heart Rate

Lactate Threshold HR = (Value 1 + Value 2 + Value 3) ÷ 3

= (_____ + _____ + _____) ÷ 3

= _____ b.p.m.

A few recommendations for taking the Talk Test:

■ If possible, use a heart-rate monitor. It will increase the accuracy of your results. (Your local health club may have one available.)

■ Test with the same activity (or fitness machine) you will be using in your training. If you use another activity, the test results will be meaningless. (Remember, your lactate threshold is specific to a particular activity.)

■ During the test, raise the intensity very slowly and be alert for the first signs of your breathing becoming irregular or conversation becoming difficult, otherwise you may overshoot and record values that are too high, invalidating your results.

Calculating the % VO$_2$ Max Your Threshold Heart Rate Represents

Calculating Your Maximum Heart Rate

Our next step is to figure out what percent of VO$_2$ max your lactate-threshold heart rate represents. To do that, we first need to calculate your maximum heart rate, your resting heart heart rate, and, ultimately, your heart rate reserve.

We already talked about calculating your maximum heart rate using the formula, 220 minus your age. With a minor change, we're going to do it the same way now. Here's the change: Women's maximum heart rates tend to run a bit higher than men's, so, to improve the accuracy of the calculations, we're going to employ two different formulas, one for each sex. Calculate your maximum heart rate in the box below:

Calculating Your Maximum Heart Rate

(for men)   220 b.p.m. - __49__ = __171__ b.p.m.

(for women)   227 b.p.m. - _____ = _____ b.p.m.

■ Remember, world-class athletes should have their maximum heart rates determined in the lab rather than using this formula.

Calculating Your Resting Heart Rate

We also need your resting heart rate. The resting heart rate is your pulse when you are just lounging around reading, resting, or relaxing. It's the rate at which your heart beats whenever there's little or no stress on the cardiovascular system. Since your resting heart rate is lowest when you are lying down and most stable when you have been at rest for a while, the best time to measure it is before getting out of bed in the morning.

For the next few days, take a 1-minute pulse count each morning when you wake up. Record the result in the box below. Then average the values to get your resting heart rate by following the instructions in the box.

For reference, most men have a resting heart rate somewhere in the neighborhood of 72 beats per minute; most women, slightly higher—around 80 b.p.m. These are average values. Actual recorded resting heart rates in one study of healthy adult males ran the gamut from 38 to 110, yielding an average of 64 b.p.m.; the *American Heart Association* accepts as normal a range of 50 to 100 b.p.m.

Calculating Your Resting Heart Rate

To determine your resting heart rate, take 1-minute pulse counts on several days before you get out of bed in the morning, then average the values:

Average Resting Heart Rate = The sum of all your values divided by the number of values you took.

Example: If you checked your pulse rate on three mornings and got counts of 69, 72, and 68, your average resting heart rate would be:

(69 + 72 + 68) ÷ 3 = 69.6, or 70 b.p.m.

Your RHR values: _____, _____, _____, _____

Average Resting Heart Rate = _____ ÷ _____

= _____ b.p.m.

Next, we need to calculate your heart rate reserve. To do that, just subtract your resting heart rate (from page 72) from your maximum heart rate (from page 71).

Calculating Your Heart Rate Reserve

= Maximum HR - Resting HR

= __*171*__ b.p.m. - _____ b.p.m.

= _____ b.p.m.

Now, finally, we can calculate the percentage of VO_2 max represented by the lactate-threshold heart rate you determined with the Talk Test. That's important because you'll be able to use the percentage to compare yourself to the rest of the world (remember, the average person has a lactate threshold at 50% of VO_2 max and endurance athletes have lactate thresholds as high as 90% of VO_2 max) and to determine your low-value exercise heart rate for LSD training.

Calculating % VO_2

To calculate your lactate threshold percentage of VO_2 max, subtract your resting heart rate from your lactate-threshold heart rate, divide the result by your heart rate reserve, and multiply by 100:

$$\% \text{ of } VO_2 \text{ Max} = \frac{\text{Lactate Threshold HR - Resting HR}}{\text{HR Reserve}} \times 100$$

For example, suppose you were a 27-year-old female with a resting heart rate of 70 b.p.m. and an lactate-threshold heart rate—determined by taking the talk test—of 150 b.p.m. That lactate-threshold heart rate would represent the following percentage of VO_2 max:

Maximum HR = 227 b.p.m. - 27 b.p.m.
= 200 b.p.m

$$\text{HR Reserve} = \text{Maximum HR} - \text{Resting HR}$$
$$= 200 \text{ b.p.m} - 70 \text{ b.p.m}$$
$$= 130 \text{ b.p.m.}$$

$$\% \text{ of VO2 Max} = \frac{\text{Lactate-Threshold HR} - \text{Resting HR}}{\text{HR Reserve}} \times 100$$

$$= \frac{150 \text{ b.p.m} - 70 \text{ b.p.m.}}{130 \text{ b.p.m.}} \times 100$$

$$= 61\%$$

Use the box below to do the calculations on yourself.

Calculating Your
Lactate Threshold % VO2 Max

Lactate Threshold HR = __143__ b.p.m. (from pg. 70)

Resting Heart Rate = __69__ b.p.m. (from pg. 72)

Heart Rate Reserve = __74__ b.p.m. (from pg. 73)

$$\% \text{ of VO2 Max} = \frac{\text{LTHR} - \text{Resting HR}}{\text{HR Reserve}} \times 100$$

$$= \frac{\underline{143} \text{ b.p.m.} - \underline{69} \text{ b.p.m.}}{\underline{74} \text{ b.p.m.}} \times 100$$

$$= \underline{43} \%$$

We're almost done. At this point we have your high-value exercise heart rate—remember, it's your lactate-threshold heart rate—and we know what percentage of VO2 max that lactate-threshold heart rate represents. All we need now is your *low-*

value exercise heart rate and we're ready to start training. You want about a 10% spread between your high- and low-exercise-heart-rate values. So we subtract 10 from the percentage of VO_2 max we just calculated, and plug this new percentage into the Karvonen formula to get a heart rate.

Let's stay with the same example we used on the last page. Our 27-year-old female would have a low-value exercise heart rate percentage of...

$$61\% - 10\% = 51\%$$

...and a low-value exercise heart rate of...

(HR Reserve $\times$ LVEHR %) + Resting HR
= (130 b.p.m. $\times$ 51%) + 70 b.p.m.
= 136 b.p.m.

Use the box below to calculate your low-value exercise HR.

Calculating Your Low-Value Exercise Heart Rate

LTHR % VO_2 Max = __143__ b.p.m. (from pg. 74)

Resting Heart Rate = __69__ b.p.m. (from pg. 72)

Heart Rate Reserve = __171__ b.p.m. (from pg. 73)

Low-Value Exercise HR % = LTHR % VO_2 Max - 10%

= __33__ % - 10%

= (HR Reserve $\times$ LVEHR %) + Resting HR

= (__171__ b.p.m. $\times$ ~~33~~%) + __69__ b.p.m.

= __126~~30~~__ b.p.m. + _____ b.p.m.

= _____ b.p.m.

126 – 143

Translating to Beats-Per-10-Seconds

One more small step. It's important to keep up your pace during VO$_2$ max work. In fact, frequent 1-minute breaks to check your heart rate would significantly decrease the effectiveness of your training. To minimize the problem, we simply convert the numbers that represent your low-value and high-value exercise heart rates to *beats-per-10-seconds* instead of beats-per-minute by dividing each by 6. With your guideline numbers converted this way, you can limit your pulse checks to 10 seconds apiece.

For example: if you came out with values of 155 and 165 beats per minute, your 10-second values would be...

$$\text{Low} = 155 \text{ b.p.m.} \div 6 = 25 \text{ beats per 10 secs.}$$
$$\text{High} = 165 \text{ b.p.m.} \div 6 = 27 \text{ beats per 10 secs.}$$

Calculating Your 10-Second Exercise Heart Rate Range

Low = _____ b.p.m. ÷ 6

= _____ b.p. 10 secs.

High = _____ b.p.m. ÷ 6

= _____ b.p. 10 secs.

And that's *really* it!

Using Your Exercise-Heart-Rate Range

In case the exercise-heart-rate range concept is new to you, let's go over how you would actually use the numbers in your training. Let's assume your exercise of choice for VO$_2$ max training is running and that this is your first day out.

You would start off at a slow-to-moderate jog. At the first hint of breathing difficulty, you would slow to a walk, locate your pulse at your wrist, and take a 10-second count. If your heart rate was above the high-value exercise heart rate, you would:

- Make a mental note of how you felt, paying particular attention to the rate and depth of your breathing.
- Continue to walk slowly and take 10-second counts.
- Note your breathing and how you felt when the count reached your high-value exercise heart rate to use as a future guide.
- Resume jogging as soon as your heart rate reached your low-value exercise heart rate.

Whenever you're using the technique, you should stop and monitor every few minutes even in the absence of obvious signs of distress. Any time your pulse is below your low-value exercise heart rate, pick up the pace. If it's within your target range, keep going at the same pace.

Warning! Always slow down and monitor at once if you suspect you might be pushing too hard—at the onset of gasping, nausea, or shortness of breath.

THE QUALITATIVE APPROACH

At the beginning of this chapter, we said that there are two common approaches to aerobic training, quantitative and qualitative. Time to dispense with all the numbers and get on to the qualitative approach.

After a month or two of carefully monitoring your pulse, you should be able to judge your upper and lower exercise heart rates by feel alone. From that point forward, you can basically dispense with the pulse checks—although we recommend you continue to monitor at least once a week to maintain the accuracy of your mental standard.

Your *ongoing* approach to LSD, then, amounts to perpetually taking the Talk Test. Whenever you train, constantly monitor your breathing and adjust your pace to remain just below the unstable ventilation threshold. That will ensure you are working at a safe and productive level for LSD.

❖   ❖   ❖

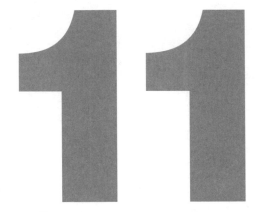

LACTATE THRESHOLD TRAINING

Almost everyone needs to do long, steady distance to establish an aerobic foundation. But if your goal is to break through to new heights of aerobic performance, you eventually need to do some threshold work as well. (Surprisingly, one of the components of threshold work can be essential if you're trying to lose weight, too. We'll see how in a moment.)

Lactate threshold training works by:

■ decreasing the amount of lactic acid you produce when exercising at a high-intensity level

■ improving your ability to buffer the lactic acid you do produce

Let's take each of the three lactate-threshold-training building blocks we defined two chapters back in turn: **threshold runs**, **intervals**, and **peaking threshold runs**.

THRESHOLD RUNS

The first building block for lactate threshold training is threshold "runs." As we said, these consist of 20- to 40-minute sessions of your chosen aerobic exercise done at your lactate threshold. (Determine the correct pace using the Talk Test described on page 69.)

Threshold runs are a "big guns" approach to raising your lactate threshold. They'll do the job quickly, but they're not fun. You need them if you're a competitive endurance athlete or if your sport requires prolonged exertion at or above the lactate threshold. Soccer, for example, involves a lot of fairly continuous, high-intensity running back and forth across a long playing field; it's a candidate for threshold-run training. Basketball, on the other hand, is not: Although you spend time running back and forth on the court, the running periods are short and they're followed by much lower-intensity periods of standing. So basketball is a candidate for high-intensity *interval* training, not threshold-run training.

Of the four main training goals we've been considering throughout **Max O2**—losing bodyfat for bodybuilding, improving general fitness, losing weight, and training for endurance events—only training for endurance events requires threshold runs.

INTERVALS

Intervals are the most flexible form of threshold training. Recall that they consist of alternating periods of activity (called **on-time**) and rest (called **off-time**); you can vary the activity and rest periods over a broad range to match your fitness and athletic requirements.

Intervals are most valuable because they allow you to train at a very high intensity—high enough to recruit the 2B fibers—without running afoul of lactic acid production. A pace that would reduce you to a lump on the ground if you tried to keep it up for five minutes straight is perfectly doable (albeit uncomfortable) when pursued in two-minute intervals with 30-second rests in between.

Long, steady distance will not produce the physiological changes necessary to elevate your lactate threshold. But high-intensity intervals will—quickly, in fact. Even a conservative interval program will elevate your lactate threshold markedly within 3 to 4 weeks.

Let's take a look at some recommendations for using intervals to condition for endurance sports and also at how they figure into losing weight.

Using Intervals to Elevate the Lactate Threshold

To improve your ability to handle lactate, total interval on-time should be at least 5, and at most 25, minutes. That means that when you add up all the time you actually spend running, swimming, or whatever (but exclude the time spent resting) the total ranges from 5 to 25 minutes. The lengths of the intervals themselves depend on your fitness goal—or, if you are an endurance athlete, on your event. Longer events, such as marathon, require longer, slower intervals; shorter events, such as a 5- or 10K, require shorter, faster ones.

Intervals are specified as a ratio. The first number corresponds to the activity period; the second, to the rest period. Training at a 5-to-1 ratio means that for every 5 minutes you work, you rest for one minute. A 3-to-2 ratio means that for every 3 minutes you work, you rest for 2. Below are some very general guidelines for using intervals as an adjunct to athletic conditioning.

Short Events

If you're training for an event shorter than a 10K, use a 2-to-1 ratio—for every minute of actual work time, rest 30 seconds. Start with a total on-time of 5 minutes, and as your fitness level improves, gradually increase to 25 minutes. Remember, the goals represent total *on-time*. That means that at the top level, 25 minutes of on-time will involve a 42½ minute workout because work periods alternate with rest periods.

Long Events

If you are training for a longer event, more than a 10K, use a 1-to-2 ratio for a total of 5 to 10 minutes of on-time. At 10 minutes of total on-time, your workout will take 30 minutes, 10 for the work and 20 for the rest.

Rest

The way you rest has a significant impact on the effectiveness of your interval training. For both short and long events, rests during interval training should be active, not passive. Walk around, bounce slowly from foot to foot or do some other low-level activity involving the muscles you are training. Don't sit or lie down. Studies show that active rest helps you recover more fully and more quickly, probably because the increased circulation associated with active rest allows more lactate to be taken up by the liver and the heart, and helps with thermal regulation (getting rid of excess heat).

Intervals can play two roles in the program of someone who's significantly overweight. The first involves your initial attempt to use exercise to drop those extra pounds.

We said earlier that the average VO_2 max runs around 40 to 50 mls/kg/min, and that lactate thresholds typically run about 50% of that. That gives our average individual the capacity to handle activities requiring up to about 25 mls/kg/min.

Now, consider someone who's so overweight and so sedentary that their VO_2 max has dropped to 20 mls/kg/min. With a lactate threshold of 50% of that, that individual is going to have a hard time with activities requiring over 10 mls/kg/min. Which means that even walking down the street or slowly pedaling an exercise bicycle will be *very* uncomfortable.

To lose weight, you need to burn at least 300 extra calories per workout, or 2000 calories a week. With a usable aerobic capacity of 10 mls/kg/min, you can't even come come close to that because you can't sustain the lowest pace of long, steady distance work. *You're basically too unfit to lose weight!*

The solution is interval training. Even someone who's very overweight can do 5, 10, maybe even 15 one-minute intervals at an intensity that will elevate both VO_2 max and lactate threshold. In a matter of weeks on an interval program, you'll be in good enough shape to burn more calories more quickly doing long, steady distance work. Here are the general guidelines for interval-based weight loss:

The goal is to burn as many calories as possible as quickly as possible, within the limits imposed by your current fitness level. So you want your intervals to be as long as possible. Start with a ratio of 1-to-1, 1 minute on, 1 minute off, and a total on-time of no more than 60 minutes. If this is too difficult, try increasing rest or decreasing intensity rather than decreasing on-time per interval. If you can exercise easily at a 1-to-1 ratio, move up to a 2-to-1 ratio (2 minutes on, 1 minute off), then a 3-to-1 ratio (3 minutes on, 1 minute off), and so on. Work up your on-time during a single interval to 15 minutes before moving on to an LSD program.

15 MIN.

A few notes to make the initial weight-loss interval period more productive. Your best bet is to use a treadmill, if you have one available. Almost everyone is more comfortable with the mechanics of walking than, say, cycling or rowing. Comfort translates into less local muscular fatigue, making your

Best Weight-Loss Activity Choices

current lactate threshold less of an impediment. Try walking with zero incline. If you can get through a beginning interval program like that, increase the pace or the incline, but not both.

If you don't have access to a treadmill (or you hate them) and you want to use a stationary bicycle instead, keep in mind that you can lower the intensity below the supposed minimum setting by turning the bike off and just pedaling with no resistance. Try that if you are have difficulty completing one-minute intervals even at the lowest setting.

Advanced Intervals for Weight Loss

We've just seen how you can use intervals to jump-start a weight-loss program. You can also use them in a second way at advanced levels for very rapid weight loss.

The key is calories. Despite all the attention given to "burning fat" during exercise, what really counts is *total calories used*. You lose weight when, on an ongoing basis, you use more calories than you consume—that's called creating a **calorie deficit**. The bigger the calorie deficit, the greater the weight loss.

High-intensity intervals allow you to burn *many* more calories in less time than LSD training, making them ideal for an advanced weight loss program. (You have to build a high level of fitness before using them, though, or you risk health complications.) We'll give detailed recommendations for an interval-based weight-loss routine in the *Program* chapter.

Intervals for Other Goals

Of the three lactate-threshold-training building blocks, only interval training is of general use to a broad spectrum of individuals. As we just said, if you're trying to lose weight, you may need intervals just to get to the point of being able to *do* long, steady distance training. Later, you can use them to burn more calories to take the weight off faster. If you're working to improve your general fitness, intervals are your ticket to quick progress. And if you're an endurance athlete, intervals allow you to tailor your training to match your event.

Only bodybuilders may not benefit from intervals. Too much high-intensity aerobic work can lead to glycogen depletion and overtraining of the Type 2 fibers, resulting in mass loss. To hold mass, it's essential to minimize recruiting the fast-twitch fiber types during aerobic training.

PEAKING THRESHOLD RUNS

If threshold runs represent a "big guns" approach to threshold training, the third building block, peaking threshold runs, is a veritable cannon. Recall that peaking threshold runs involve various combinations of intervals and threshold runs. As with regular threshold runs, you can do a peaking threshold "run" with any aerobic activity.

No getting around it, these hurt! In fact, they're so intense that you only want to use them once per week, or once every other week. Still, peaking threshold runs are the most effective way to maximize the speed of lactate clearance. They prepare you for that track or cycling opponent who breaks away from the pack, forcing you to sprint to keep up *and then quickly re-establish a steady rate.* They're also useful for martial artists or boxers. Both are constantly forced to launch a flurry of blows from a near-threshold intensity level, then drop back and defend without much time to recover.

Bodybuilders and individuals trying to lose weight or get fit do not need to do peaking threshold runs.

APPLICABILITY OF THRESHOLD-TRAINING BUILDING BLOCKS FOR VARIOUS GOALS

	INTERVALS	THRESHOLD RUNS	PEAKING THRESHOLD RUNS
BODY-BUILDING	Avoid	Avoid	Avoid
WEIGHT LOSS	Yes, for extremely low fitness levels and advanced weight-loss programs	Not necessary	Not necessary
GENERAL FITNESS	Optional	Optional	Optional
ATHLETIC ENDURANCE	Yes, depending on sport	Yes, depending on sport	Yes, depending on sport

❖   ❖   ❖

12

THE PROGRAMS: HOW MUCH, HOW OFTEN

In the last two chapters, we looked at single instances of using each of the **Max O$_2$** building blocks. Now let's see how you schedule them over weeks, even months, to create the optimum aerobics training programs for bodybuilding fat loss, improving general fitness, losing weight, and conditioning for endurance sports.

THE F.I.T.T. TRAINING MODEL

To create a weekly or monthly schedule, you specify how much and how often to use any of the building blocks in terms of four variables...

■ **Frequency**
■ **Intensity** (also called *pace*)
■ **Time** (also called *duration*)
■ **Type** (also called *mode*)

Frequency

Frequency is the number of times per day or week you use a particular building block—for example, doing long, steady distance training 4 times per week or intervals 3 times per week.

Intensity

Intensity is how hard you train during each session. It's often stated in terms of percent of VO2 max or some measure of *distance-per-unit-time*, such as miles-per-hour or steps-per-minute. But, as explained in Chapter 10, you can match intensity recommendations to your personal fitness level more exactly by specifying intensity in relation to lactate-threshold heart rate (LTHR).

Time

Time is how long you keep at a particular exercise: for instance, doing long, steady distance for *20 minutes*, using an interval on-time of *5 minutes*.

Type

And *type* is the exercise you use for any of the four building blocks. Type could be running, swimming, cycling, or any other aerobic activity.

Combining all four variables, we might specify your LSD schedule for a particular week by saying you should:

- train once per day for 6 days (frequency)
- stay below your lactate threshold heart rate (intensity)
- work for 20 to 40 minutes per session (time)
- use running as your exercise (type)

Packaging

There's one more element we'll be dealing with below that isn't part of the F.I.T.T. model—**packaging.** Packaging is the integration of the **Max O2** building for a particular program or goal. When you start combining different training elements, you can't just add all the individual F.I.T.T. requirements together or you'll quickly exceed the limits of reasonable training volume. Exceeding those limits increases both your risk of injury and likelihood of overtraining.

To maintain a reasonable training volume, you have to do two things:

- Decrease the amount of (or time devoted to) one building block as you schedule in others. For example, where the stand-alone recommendations for LSD for general fitness call for 5 to 6 training days per week, we drop that to 4 to 5 days per week once we add a day of intervals.

■ Monitor, and adjust for, overtraining. Do that by checking your pulse every morning as described on page 70. If it's 10% above normal, decrease your training intensity for that day (for example, if you've scheduled an interval day, do an LSD day instead). If it's 20% above normal, take a day off.*

These guidelines only apply once you've established a consistent resting-pulse baseline. If you're a beginner and your resting pulse remains elevated for a week or more without your resuming training—and you're not experiencing undo life stress—you may have simply have miscalculated or mismeasured your resting pulse rate in the first place. Establish a new baseline, resume training, and begin monitoring again.

Different F.I.T.T.s for Different Goals

Each of our four main goals—bodybuilding fat loss, improved fitness, weight loss, and increased athletic endurance—requires different values for the F.I.T.T. variables for each of the applicable building blocks.

In fact, each of those training goals calls for different *sets* of F.I.T.T. exercise prescriptions for different times of the year. Bodybuilding, for example, typically requires more time for aerobic training during the two months before a contest than at other times. The first three programs that follow—for bodybuilding, general fitness, and weight loss—detail both the optimum F.I.T.T. recommendations for each goal and the way those programs should vary over time; the fourth (for endurance training) lays out a framework on which you can build a custom program. It's beyond the scope of any book to lay out full schedules for all individuals for all endurance sports, given the specificity that must be built into such routines.

Before proceeding, take the Talk Test to determine your lactate-threshold heart rate (LTHR). All the programs below use that value to establish an exercise-heart-rate range based on your current fitness level. For LSD, you will usually be directed to work in a range starting *at* your LTHR and ranging *down* 10%. For threshold runs, you will be directed to work in a range starting at your LTHR and ranging *up* 10%, and for intervals above threshold, you will be directed to work in a

---

*This doesn't apply to bodybuilders in the final weeks of contest preparation, whose regimens may wreak havoc with their resting and training heart rates.

range starting *10 beats higher than your LTHR* and ranging *up 10%* from there.

On to the programs!

AEROBIC TRAINING FOR BODYBUILDERS

The bodybuilder's program will involve two phases, **ongoing** and **pre-contest**.

We already have Rule #1 for both phases: *No high-intensity work!* No intervals, no threshold runs, no peaking threshold runs. And, for that matter, no LSD anywhere close to your lactate threshold. For bodybuilding fat loss, you should use a heart rate about 15 b.p.m. *lower* than your Talk Test heart rate as the *ceiling* for LSD work. That will ensure you stay below the lactate threshold.

Rule #2, which applies mainly to the pre-contest phase, is: *burn as many calories as possible without disregarding Rule #1.* That means the more, the longer, the better—but still at a low intensity. Set an upper weight-loss limit of one to two pounds per week. Faster fat loss will likely be accompanied by lean tissue loss, as well. Translating that into numbers, you should aim to create about a 750-calorie *deficit* per day through combined dietary and exercise adjustment. **Limit your dietary calorie adjustment to a reduction of no more than 200 to 300 calories per day** or you will trigger the body's tendency to become more fuel efficient in the face of decreased caloric intake *and you won't lose the fat you want to.* That leaves about 450 to 550 calories to burn via LSD. You'll easily burn that many by cycling or running on a treadmill for an hour at 50% to 60% of VO_2 max. Above all, make sure you allow enough time before competition to lose all the weight you need to at the one to two pound-per-week rate so you don't get into trouble with glycogen depletion and overtraining!

One last point. Although you burn more fat the longer your LSD session, you'll burn more *calories* overall during two short sessions that total *more time* (assuming the same intensity on all counts). Remember: Total calories burned during exercise has a greater effect on fat loss than total fat burned. For the bodybuilder, that means that if you don't have the energy to go for an hour to an a 1½ hours straight on the exercise bike (perhaps because you're on a pre-contest, calorie-restricted diet), you should break your daily LSD work into 2 or 3 half-hour sessions, rather than doing one session that results in decreased total LSD time. All other factors being equal, you'll lose more fat that way.

Here's the specific program. Note the different recommendations for ongoing vs. pre-contest training.

Frequency

- **Ongoing:** 1 session per day, 3 to 4 days per week
- **Pre-Contest:** 1 to 2 sessions per day, 6 to 7 days per week

Intensity

- Below lactate threshold (usually around 50% to 60% of VO$_2$ max)

Time

- **Ongoing:** 15 minutes to 1 hour per day, (workouts approaching an hour can be performed in two sessions)
- **Pre-Contest:** 1 hour to 1½ hours per day, (can be performed in two or three sessions)

Type

- The physical shock from weight-bearing aerobic exercises such as jogging or jumping rope combined with extended high-intensity resistance work tends to promote overtraining even at low aerobic exercise intensities. As a result, you're better off using *non*-weight bearing aerobic exercise such as stationary cycling for your fat-loss program.

- Also, as mentioned earlier, studies show that swimming produces less fat loss for any given caloric expenditure than other aerobic exercises, probably due to the coldness of the water. Avoid swimming as well.

Progression

- If you are very out of shape, begin with the LSD recommendations for the initial stage of the *General Fitness* program below. Use that program until you can perform the minimum level of LSD training specified here. Remember to keep intensity well below threshold at all times!

Notes for Pre-Contest Training

■ Aim to create a calorie deficit of about 750 calories per day, achieving no more than 200 to 300 calories of deficit through dietary restriction

■ Limit aerobic work to what results in a maximum of 1 to 2 lbs. of fat loss per week

None.

Lactate-Threshold Training

You don't *need* threshold training to get fit; LSD alone will do the job. But since adding even a little high-intensity work to a general fitness LSD program will produce more rapid progress, we provide an optional interval workout after the LSD-only program below. *The optional threshold training is intended for individuals who have worked through the **initial** and **improvement** stages of the General Fitness program below, or who are already highly fit.*

AEROBIC TRAINING FOR GENERAL FITNESS

There are three stages to the **Max O₂** General Fitness program: an **initial** stage, an **improvement** stage, and a **maintenance** stage.

The initial stage lasts 4 to 6 weeks, depending on how fit you are to begin with. During this stage, keep intensity low and time short.

Next comes the improvement stage. This usually lasts 12 to 20 weeks, but can last much longer. Here, strive to burn a full 300 calories per exercise bout. As you work through this phase, increase frequency, intensity or time every week (or every other week, if you're in really poor shape to begin with)—but *never* raise more than one at a time. Work up to the upper end of the time range before beginning to raise frequency or intensity, following the *progression* guidelines listed below.

After you've reached your desired fitness level, you move on to the maintenance stage. Research indicates that you can maintain your aerobic capacity even if you substantially decrease the *frequency* of your workouts (down to a minimum of 2 days

LSD

a week)—as long as you keep *intensity* at your previous peak level. The reverse isn't true. Decreasing *intensity* even a little quickly results in a substantial loss of aerobic capacity.

LSD

The Initial Stage (4 to 6 Weeks)

Frequency

■ 1 session per day, 3 to 6 days per week

Intensity

■ Below lactate threshold—use Talk Test heart rate as the *ceiling* for your exercise-heart-rate range. Tend toward the *low end* of the range at first. Try to be operating at the upper end of the range by the fourth or fifth week.

Time

■ 12 to 15 minutes to start; 20 to 30 minutes by the end of the initial phase

Type

■ Whatever aerobic exercise you enjoy. We recommend staying away from stair-stepping machines at this stage because their high anaerobic demand may limit your ability to complete your LSD sessions.

Progression

■ Work up from the low values specified above to the high values, systematically increasing *time* to the high value before beginning to increase intensity.

LSD

The Improvement Phase (12 to 20 Weeks)

Frequency

■ 1 session per day, 3 to 6 days per week

Intensity

■ At or below lactate threshold—use the Talk Test heart rate as the *ceiling* for your exercise-heart-rate range. Train at the upper end of the range.

Time

■ 20 to 60 minutes

Type

■ Whatever aerobic exercise you enjoy

Progression

■ Work up from the low values specified above to the high values, systematically increasing your time to the high value before beginning to increase intensity.

■ Limit *time* increases to no more than 10% to 20% per week. For example, if you were running for 20 minutes, the maximum acceptable time increase would be anywhere from 20 minutes + 10%, or 22 minutes, to 20 minutes + 20%, or 24 minutes.

■ Limit *frequency* increases to no more than one additional day per week.

■ Only raise one F.I.T.T. variable at a time.

Frequency

■ 1 to 2 times per week

Intensity

■ Above lactate threshold—use the Talk Test heart rate as the *floor* for your exercise-heart-rate range.

Time

■ 3-to-1 ratio: from 1 minute of on-time and 20 seconds of off-time to 3 minutes of on-time and 1 minute of off-time

■ Total on-time to range from 9 to 27 minutes

Type

■ The same aerobic exercise you use for LSD work

Progression

■ Begin with 2 to 3 intervals. Add 1 interval per week until you reach the maximum.

Intervals (Optional)

Packaging, as we said, is the integration of the **Max O$_2$** building blocks for a particular program or goal. Remember that as you add days for performance of one **Max O$_2$** building block,

Packaging

you decrease the time allotted for another. Here's how to integrate LSD and intervals for general fitness:

- Instead of 4 to 6 days of LSD, do 3 to 5 days of LSD plus 1 day of above-lactate-threshold intervals.

— or —

- Do 3 to 4 days of LSD plus 2 days of above-lactate threshold intervals.
- Do not do LSD and interval training on the same days.

AEROBIC TRAINING FOR WEIGHT LOSS

Aerobic training for weight loss is similar to aerobic training for general fitness, with three important differences. First, as we mentioned earlier, many people who are very overweight are also very underfit—enough so that even the initial stage in the General Fitness Program will be more intense than they can handle. To provide a bridge from totally sedentary to minimally fit, the weight-loss program includes a special "pre-initial" stage of intervals. This stage lasts as long as it takes to build the fitness necessary to do 15 minutes of uninterrupted, low-intensity LSD training. (If you can already do 15 minutes of LSD, you can skip the pre-initial stage.)

The second difference between the weight-loss and general fitness programs involves exercise *type*. Where the general fitness program calls for any aerobic exercise you enjoy, the weight-loss model recommends using *weight-bearing* exercises such as walking or jogging. Studies suggest that weight-bearing activities promote faster caloric expenditure. Which means weight-bearing activities may increase your aerobic efficiency more rapidly than non-weight bearing ones.

That's just what you want for weight loss. You want to get as aerobically efficient (and aerobically fit) as quickly as possible so you can expend more calories more quickly. The more calories expended, the faster the weight loss (assuming you're not offsetting the extra expenditure by eating an extra pint of Häagen Dazs every night).

The third difference is that, where 20 minutes 3 times a week is sufficient to improve general fitness, it's insufficient—or at least far from optimum—for weight loss. Once you're fit enough to handle long workouts, you want total LSD durations of an hour to an hour-and-a-half per day at the highest intensity you can stand. For even faster weight loss, you can use above-threshold intervals. As recommended for fat loss for bodybuilders, you should split your LSD workout into several shorter sessions if that means you can increase total LSD time per day. Remember—total calories burned is the most important variable for weight loss. (See the box below for a comparison of the effects of different durations and intensities on fat loss.)

The **Max O2** weight-loss program begins on the next page.

EFFECTS OF DURATION AND INTENSITY ON FAT LOSS

To be sure you're clear on the interaction between fuel burned and calories used, let's consider a few comparisons:

- Given a low-intensity, 40-minute workout that burns 120 calories and a high-intensity, 40-minute workout that burns 250, the high-intensity workout will make a greater contribution to losing weight—*because of the higher caloric expenditure.*

- Given a high-intensity, 20-minute workout that burns 200 calories and a low-intensity, 40-minute workout that burns 150, the shorter, high-intensity workout will make a greater contribution to losing weight—*again, because of the higher caloric expenditure.*

- Given a high-intensity, 20-minute workout that burns 200 calories and a low-intensity, 40-minute workout that *also* burns 200 calories, the longer workout is better. Since the most important factor—calories burned—is the same on both counts, we look to other variables to determine the better choice. In this case, it's workout intensity. Longer, low-intensity workouts burn less glycogen, resulting in more rapid post-workout recovery, higher post-workout energy levels, and a lower post-workout appetite. They also burn more fat, although fuel burned during exercise is actually the least important consideration for weight loss.

Pre-Initial Stage
Intervals

Frequency

- 6 to 7 days per week

Intensity

- As low as possible (try to stay below your lactate-threshold heart rate if possible)

Time (Work-to-Rest Ratio)

- From 1-to-1 (1 minute of on-time, 1 minute of off-time) to 15-to-1 (15 minutes of on-time, 1 minute of off-time)
- Total on-time to range from 1 to 15 minutes

Type

- Preferably weight-bearing aerobic activities such as walking or jogging (unless extreme overweight makes weight-bearing exercise painful for the joints, in which case you should use non-weight-bearing activities, such as cycling)

Progression

- Begin with 2 to 3 intervals. Add 1 to 2 intervals per session up to 15 minutes on-time, then start increasing the work/rest ratio as quickly as you comfortably can (increase from 1-to-1, to 2-to-1, to 3-to-1, and so on until you eventually can do a single, uninterrupted "interval" 15 minutes long.

LSD

LSD
Initial Stage
(4 to 6 Weeks)

Frequency

- 1 session per day, 3 to 5 days per week

Intensity

- Below lactate threshold—use Talk Test heart rate as the *ceiling* for your exercise-heart-rate range. Tend toward the *low end* of the range.

Time

- 12 to 15 minutes to start

- 20 to 30 minutes by the end of the initial stage

Type

- Preferably weight-bearing aerobic activities

Progression

- Work up from the low frequency, time, and intensity values specified above to the high values, systematically increasing *time* to the highest time value before beginning to increase intensity. Limit time increases to 10% to 20% per week and frequency increases to 1 day a week.

Frequency

- 1 session per day, 3 to 6 days per week

Intensity

- At or below lactate threshold—use Talk Test heart rate as the *ceiling* for your exercise heart rate range. Train at the upper end of the range.

Time

- 20 to 120 minutes; may be broken up into 2 or 3 shorter sessions per day

Type

- Preferably weight-bearing activities

Progression

- Same as above. Work up from the low values specified above to the high values, systematically increasing *time* to the high value before beginning to increase intensity. Limit increases to 10% to 20% per week and frequency increases to 1 day a week.

D on't try advanced intervals until you've completed three months of LSD-only training or you're comfortable doing 60 minutes of continuous LSD work.

LSD
___

Improvement Phase (12 to 20 Weeks)

Advanced Intervals (Optional)

Frequency

- 1 to 5 times per week

Intensity

- At lactate threshold—use the Talk Test heart rate as your exercise heart rate.

Time (Work-to-Rest Ratio)

- **To start:** 1-to-1.5 (from 30 seconds of on-time, 45 seconds of off-time up to 5 minutes of on-time, 7.5 minutes of off-time)
- **Very Advanced:** 1-to-1 (from 30 seconds of on-time, 30 seconds of off-time up to 5 minutes of on-time, 5 minutes of off-time)
- Total on-time to range from 30 minutes to 75 minutes

AEROBIC TRAINING FOR ENDURANCE ATHLETES

Endurance athletes participate in a class of sports called **aerobic sports** (see list below). Aerobic sports involve sustained effort with only minor changes in speed or direction; they require a high VO$_2$ max and a high lactate threshold. Although there are definite differences in the performance demands for each of these sports, you can use the following

AEROBIC SPORTS

- Cross-Country Skiing
- Rowing—long distance
- Backpacking
- Bicycling
- Running
- Distance Skating
- Snowshoeing
- Swimming
- Walking
- Triathalons

guidelines as a framework on which to build a custom training regimen. Remember to be as specific to your sport as possible—and keep in mind that "specificity" applies to more than just the type of sport—you must also consider duration, distance, terrain changes, thermal demands, and so on.

LSD

Frequency
- 2 to 7 days per week

Intensity
- Below lactate threshold

Time
- 20 to 120 minutes

Threshold Runs

Frequency
- 0 to 2 days per week

Intensity
- At lactate threshold

Time
- 20 to 40 minutes

Intervals

Frequency
- 0 to 3 days per week

Intensity
- Above lactate threshold

Time (Work-to-Rest Ratio)
- 1-to-1 (from 30 seconds of on-time, 30 seconds of off-time up to 5 minutes of on-time, 5 minutes of off-time)
- 1-to-1.5 (from 30 seconds of on-time, 45 seconds of off-time up to 5 minutes of on-time, 7.5 minutes of off-time)
- Total on-time to range from 5 to 30 minutes

Peaking Threshold Runs

Frequency

- 1 day every week or every other week

Intensity

- **Intervals**—On-time intensity should be set higher than your lactate threshold; off-time (rest) intensity should be well below your lactate threshold, but above resting level.
- **Threshold Run**—at your lactate threshold

Time

- **Intervals**—3 to 10 minutes of *total* on-time
- 1-to-1 (from 30 seconds of on-time, 30 seconds of off-time up to 5 minute of on-time, 5 minutes of off-time)
- 1-to-1.5 (from 30 seconds of on-time, 45 seconds of off-time up to 5 minute of on-time, 7.5 minutes of off-time)
- **Threshold**—20 to 40 minutes

Peaking Threshold Run Packaging

Start with 3 intervals followed by a 20-minute threshold session once every 2 weeks. As your condition improves, you can add more intervals and/or increase the length of the threshold session to meet the needs of your specific sport.

Monthly and Yearly Packaging

It's beyond the scope of this book to lay out full year-round programs, or **periodization schedules,** for all the building blocks for each aerobic sport. The most important concept to keep in mind when doing so for yourself is matching type of training to nature of sport.

That does it for the basic **Max O$_2$** programs!

You can use these programs with almost any type of aerobic training. By far the most popular activities are running, walking, swimming, and cycling, all of which have been the subject of countless books and articles. In the remainder of the *Training* section, though, we present specific programs for two very effective aerobic exercises—slideboarding and jumping rope—about which relatively little has been written. Also, we offer a survey of the most popular types of stationary ergometers, considering their benefits and drawbacks and suggesting ways to use them to maximum advantage.

❖   ❖   ❖

13

ERGOMETER TRAINING

Most gyms offer a wide variety of aerobic equipment options—steppers, bikes, and treadmills, just to name a few. As these devices—called **ergometers**—become more and more popular, many questions arise: Is indoor training as good as outdoor training? How does ergometer training compare to aerobic dance? What's the best ergometer to use to meet my goals? How do I maximize my results on a particular ergometer?

In this chapter, we'll cover the general advantages and disadvantages of stationary ergometers, comparing them to other forms of training. We'll also take a look at types of ergometers and discuss how to choose the right machine for your training goals. Finally, we'll look at key training points for specific machines.

STATIONARY ERGOMETERS VS. OUTDOOR TRAINING

In general, ergometers offer the advantages of **control**, **adjustability**, and **ease of monitoring**.

Where outdoor training leaves you little control over things like the steepness of a grade or weather conditions, indoor ergometer training allows you to work in a sheltered, predictable environment, where the demands of the "course" are fully adjustable. And unlike outdoor forms of training, most ergometers provide valuable information about your workout, including cadence, distance covered, grade, speed, and (though not 100% accurate) caloric expenditure.

Whether these and other ergometer features are advantages or disadvantages depends on your training goals and tastes. Some people *like* their constancy, but many athletes find that ergometers' lack of variability makes it difficult to use them to prepare for outdoor competition. Likewise, some people consider ergometers monotonous. But others who feel bored by *any* form of exercise find ergometer training the most workable choice—because you can read or watch TV while using them.

Since ergometer training is, by and large, an indoor activity, it invites comparison to the other major indoor aerobic activity—**aerobic dance** in all its forms, including high impact, low impact, hip-hop, and step. Here as well, the advantages of ergometer training center on the greater control they provide over intensity and progression, and on their detailed monitoring capabilities. Let's explore these points.

ERGOMETER TRAINING VS. AEROBIC DANCE

A 1-hour aerobic class may only provide about 45 minutes of work within the exercise-heart-rate range, thanks to a format that tries to incorporate flexibility and toning work as well. Ergometers, however, offer an aerobic workout that is 100% aerobic.

Intensity

Most aerobic dance movements are limited in the degree to which they can be made progressively more difficult—a necessary factor, if the workout is to continue to be effective. While you might try kicking a little higher, or raising the height of your step platform, or even taking more classes per week, aerobic dance cannot match the machine's ability to provide a constantly increasing load. (Since aerobic dance is a weight-bearing activity, increasing the number of classes also increases your risk of injury. Jolting-type aerobic dance—step, high-impact, etc.—should not be performed more than 3 to 5 times per week.)

Progression

Monitoring Facility

In addition to other useful data, the ergometer provides detailed feedback concerning your *pace*. Monitoring your pace is key to getting the most effective workout possible. In an aerobic dance class, you will naturally kick higher and harder on some days than on others, and there is no external feedback to tell you just how hard you worked. Also, most aerobic dance classes are too intense for LSD training, sending participants beyond their lactate thresholds many times during the class. The ergometer allows you to pace your workout with precision for the fastest possible results.

On the other hand, since *consistency* may be the single most important aspect of any training regimen, you shouldn't overlook the benefits from the social aspects of aerobic dance. Aerobics classes offer a camaraderie and a sense of belonging that you just don't get with stationary ergometer training.

ERGOMETERS: GENERAL GUIDELINES

Today's marketplace presents the prospective stationary equipment user with a bewildering range of choices. Sure, every manufacturer claims you'll get great aerobic and weight-loss benefits from their product. But is one ergometer really the best?

Choose What You'll Use

Simply—the best piece of equipment for aerobic conditioning and weight loss is the one you *use*. Any advantage one piece of equipment has over another is for naught if you don't like the activity or find the machine uncomfortable. So make the following discussion a starting point but let personal taste be your guide. If you like two or three different activities equally, choose the one with the highest rate of caloric expenditure.

Motivational vs. Non-Motivational

Ergometers can be classified generally into two groups: **motivational** and **non-motivational**. The motivational ones force you to keep up—if you don't, either *you* fall off or *they* stop. These include treadmills, stair steppers, and climbers. Non-motivational machines, on the other hand, allow you to drift between a fast and slow pace with little or no consequence (other than perhaps a warning light). These include bicycles, arm crankers, rowers, and cross-country skiers. Non-motivational equipment requires more discipline on your part and greater attention to your workout.

To further compare types of ergometers (treadmills, rowers, etc.), we must approach them from the standpoint of our specific training goals—general fitness, weight loss, bodybuilding, or cross-training for a sport.

The Goal's the Thing

For improving general fitness, any form of ergometer that involves large muscle groups performing rhythmic movements will do the job.

These include (in descending order):

■ Cross-Country Skier

■ Treadmill

■ Bicycle

■ Stair Stepper

■ Rower

General Fitness

For losing weight, as well as improving general fitness, ergometers that make demands on large muscle mass are your best bets (see list above). Spreading the workload over a larger area causes less localized muscle fatigue. As a result, large muscle mass activities feel easier at any given workload and have a higher rate of caloric expenditure than exercises using a smaller muscle mass.

For example, arm cranking is performed by a relatively small muscle mass, making it difficult (due to local fatigue) to burn many calories. In comparison, cross-country skiing spreads the workload over a very large muscle mass and can be performed at a much higher work rate (with less fatigue), thereby burning substantially more calories.

Weight Loss

Although a bodybuilder's *method* of training will differ from that of an overweight person or someone working to improve general fitness (see Chapter 12), the criteria for choosing an appropriate machine is the same. Bodybuilders should select from the machines offering the greatest muscle involvement.

Bodybuilding

If you want to use ergometers to cross-train for a specific sport, understand that the athletic carryover of most ergometers is poor, for several reasons:

Endurance Sport Supplemental Training

The first has to do with the non-athletic body mechanics of most machines. With the exception of some rowers, your limbs work against a machine's resistance, while your torso hardly moves at all. This is quite different from the demands of most sports, in which your limbs must *propel* your torso against gravity. In addition, the athlete must face environmental factors—weather, terrain changes, and subtle variations in training surface—that ergometer training, for the most part, fails to take into account. Due to this lack of proprioceptive feedback (especially during incline work), ergometer training should not be the foundation of an athletic program, although it can be a useful addition to one.

Even when you use ergometer training in a supplementary role, observe the specificity concept and *choose stationary equipment that makes the same types of demands as the sport for which you're training*. Although non-specific training can help you accomplish goals such as weight loss, training for sports performance requires a sports-specific approach. If your event involves running, use a treadmill; if it involves rowing, use a rower, and so on. Remember, there's very little aerobic carryover from one aerobic activity to another.

KEY TRAINING POINTS FOR SPECIFIC EQUIPMENT

This section covers the merits of the individual types of machines and offers some training tips for their use. But before we look at particular machines, there are two general points to make about ergometers in relation to LSD training. The first concerns ergometer programs, the second, automatic pacing options.

Program Modes and LSD Training

Most ergometers offer several program modes (hill profile, random, etc.) that creates a workout of varying intensity. This feature is not appropriate for LSD training. Remember, LSD requires a consistent workload—but if the machine intensity is changing, your workload won't be consistent. You'll be doing intervals...not long, *steady* distance! Furthermore, program modes offer no way to set the intensity or length of individual work or rest intervals. There's also a problem with program modes as they relate to progression. If the machine picks an intensity at random, it is impossible to duplicate the settings for the next workout (let alone increase them by 10%). The best approach is to use manual mode for all your training. That way, you can increase or decrease the intensity as needed to meet your goals.

Here's the second general problem: Some ergometers have a computer-simulated pacer for you to compete against during aerobic training. Although excellent for intervals, this opponent can force you to train too hard during LSD-based workouts. When you do LSD, you need to pay attention to your body (not the computer) and maintain a conversational pace.

OK. Now we're going to list the advantages and disadvantages of the more popular ergometers and offer some training tips for their use.

Machine-based stair stepping has many things to recommend it. It provides an excellent aerobic workout and, due to its partial weight-bearing nature, improves balance and coordination.

- **Low impact / low injury.** Training on a stair climber, you are far less vulnerable to the strained knees and twisted ankles that can result from the impact of actual stair climbing.
- **Convenience**. A stair stepper saves you the chore of finding a stairway with enough stairs to provide a good workout.

- **No true step.** When climbing stairs, the muscles must overcome gravity, but with stepping machines you remain level as the machine sinks with each step. As a result, machine stepping does not improve coordination or balance to the same degree.

    Furthermore, because your body does not elevate, you can't use standard calculations to determine caloric expenditure based on step height. Manufacturers have developed their own proprietary formulas designed to offer the closest approximations possible. But to obtain reasonably accurate caloric expenditure

Computer Pacer and LSD Training

Stair Steppers (vs. Actual Stairs)

Advantages

Disadvantages

values, you have to stair step correctly, according to the guidelines listed below.

Training Points

- **Find a comfortable step height.**
- **Don't bounce off the bottom.** Bouncing at the bottom of each step creates a significant impact and can lead to injuries of the knee and spine.
- **Vary the use of your arms.** The intensity of any workload can be modified by varying how you carry your arms—either swinging, as in walking (more difficult), or hands on hips (easier).
- **Keep your hands off the rails!** Machine stepping is a partial weight-bearing activity, and the equipment uses your body weight to make its caloric calculations. *Supporting any portion of your weight on the rails will throw these calculations off.* In an informal study, we placed a heart-rate monitor on several people as they stepped at a constant intensity, first with the hands free and then while holding the rail. The results of this experiment showed that even when the rails were held lightly (for balance only) the heart rate dropped by 15% to 20%!

  With this in mind, you can see that the typical way the machine is used (set to the upper levels, elbows locked, wrists turned backwards, and feet moving at 50 mph) is not very effective. Although doing this yields a display of higher numbers of floors climbed and calories burned, the numbers are meaningless.

  Leaning on the rails can also cause various injuries to the shoulder, elbow, and wrist, including rotator cuff damage, elbow tendonitis, carpal tunnel syndrome, and ganglion cyst formation at the wrist and hand. Many physicians and physical therapists actually recommend against using stair climbers because of the injuries that can result from their misuse. But performed hands-free, stair climbing is quite safe. (Although you may occasionally need to use the rails for balance when first learning to step, work toward being hands-free as quickly as possible.)

The climbing simulator is a relative newcomer to the aerobic training arena. It is similar in effect to the stair stepper, and most of the comments made about stair steppers apply to climbers as well, with the following additions:

■ **More generalized muscle involvement.** Climbers allow the upper body to contribute to the production of force.

■ **Unilateral arm movement.** This is more of an oddity than a real disadvantage. For some reason, most climbers are designed so that your arms and legs are forced to move unilaterally, i.e., left leg with left arm. Since this is contrary to the way the body normally moves in most situations, it may feel strange at first.

■ **Less balance.** Since you hold on with your arms during climbing, your balance and coordination improves less than with hands-free stair steppers.

Rowing is an excellent non-impact, aerobic activity you can use for several training goals.

■ **Convenience and cost.** For many people, rowing a real boat is simply not an option.

■ **Very poor carryover to athletic training.** With one exception,* machine-based rowers are not mechanically specific enough to be used as a substitute for actual rowing. But they are fine for general fitness and weight loss.

Climbers

Advantages

Disadvantages

Rowers (vs. Water Rowing)

Advantages

Disadvantages

---

*the *Concept II*

Training Points

- **Use your legs, not your lower back.** Rowing can stress the lower back if you do it with improper form. To minimize low back stress, start with your legs bent and your arms straight, push back with your legs, and finish by pulling through with your arms.
- **Maintain a comfortable pace.**

Treadmills (vs. Outdoor Running)

Treadmills have been around for a long time and can be found in gyms, hospitals, and therapy units. The physical demands made by treadmill walking and running are very similar to those of their outdoor counterparts, except for incline work (see below).

Advantages

- **Adjustability of grade and speed.** Unlike outdoor running, where you have to consider the grade and distance of your route, treadmills allow you complete control of all factors affecting training intensity.

Disadvantages

- **Incline work not as specific.** The mathematical formulas for *level* treadmill work have a high correlation to outdoor activity. But the absence of the need to overcome gravity makes treadmill incline work easier than its outdoor equivalent.

Training Point

- **Don't hold the rail.** Many studies have shown that holding the rail decreases heart rate and caloric expenditure. Holding the rail can also have a negative effect on stride mechanics of walking and running.

Arm Ergometers

One of the lesser known aerobic devices, the arm ergometer is essentially a stationary bicycle, mounted so that you can turn the pedals with your arms.

Advantages

- **Upper-body endurance training.** For athletes who need upper-body endurance (wrestlers, martial artists, boxers, etc....), arm cranking is an excellent form of upper-body lactate-threshold training.

■ **Substitute training mode during lower-body rehabilitation.** Although for most people, arm ergometers are not as effective as lower-body equipment for overall aerobic conditioning, they can be an excellent means of maintaining cardiovascular fitness during rehabilitation of a lower-body injury.

■ **Not appropriate for LSD training.** Arm cranking recruits little muscle mass, making LSD training difficult.

Disadvantages

■ **Calculate a different maximum heart rate.** Due to the small muscle mass and vascular bed of the arms, adjust your usual maximum heart rate *down* by approximately 13 beats when arm cranking. Example: A 30-year-old male has a predicted maximum heart rate of 190 beats per minute (220 b.p.m. - age = Max HR). Subtract an additional 13 points to find the maximum heart rate for arm ergometry (190 b.p.m. - 13 = 177 b.p.m.).

Training Points

■ **Adjust seat height.** When the seat is properly adjusted, the uppermost position of the crank should be no higher then the level of your nose.

■ **Maintain good posture.**

The cross-country skier is the aerobic ergometer champion when it comes to VO2 max and rate of caloric expenditure. Cross-country skiers recruit both upper- and lower-body muscles, thereby spreading the workload over a large muscle mass. This wide dispersion of force means less localized muscle fatigue, allowing you to burn more calories than most other ergometers.

Cross-Country Skiers (vs. Outdoor Cross-Country Skiing)

■ **Convenience.** Indoor simulators offer year-round training in comfortable, temperate conditions.

Advantages

■ **Lack of variety.** Like other stationary ergometers, cross-country skiers don't provide the subtle vari-

Disadvantages

ations in training surface so vital to improved athletic performance.

- **Poor athletic crossover.** Only the Nordictrack cross-country ski simulators come close to matching the biomechanics of outdoor cross-country skiing.

Stationary Bicycles (vs. Outdoor Cycling)

Due to its relatively low cost and excellent cardiovascular benefits, stationary cycling has become one of the most popular forms of ergometer training.

Advantages

- **Convenience and safety.** With a stationary bike, you don't have to spend a lot of extra effort dodging cars.
- **Non-weight bearing activity.** Provides a way for extremely overweight individuals to exercise with less risk of knee injury than they might experience from high-impact weight-bearing activities.

Disadvantages

- **Potential knee strain.** Some existing knee conditions are exacerbated by cycling of any kind.

Training Points

- **Proper Seat Height.** To adjust seat height, sit on the bike with your heel on the pedal. Start pedaling at a very slow pace. The seat height is correct when the knee is just short of locked at the bottom position.
- **Proper Foot Placement.** Place the ball of your foot—not your heel—on the pedal. Pedaling with the heel can lead to injury.
- **Cadence.** To minimize knee strain, keep your cadence at 80 rpm or higher. Note: Not all stationary bicycles have a cadence function. If yours does not, use the following technique to determine your cadence: At random times during your workout, take a 15-second count of the number of times your right (or left) foot hits the bottom of the stroke and multiply by 4 to determine your revolutions per minute. If you're pedaling too slowly, lower the tension and increase your speed. After a few workouts, you'll develop a feel for the proper cadence and won't need to take a count as often.

■ Although some of the newer *Lifecycle* models do display cadence, they still calculate your caloric expenditure as though you were moving at a constant 80 rpm, regardless of your actual speed. Nevertheless, pedaling at a higher rpm is considerably more difficult and burns many more calories. Example: When pedaling in manual mode at Level 1 at a cadence of 110 rpm, the caloric expenditure is somewhere between Level 2 or level 3 at
80 rpm.

❖   ❖   ❖

14 SLIDEBOARD TRAINING

Originally designed for off-season training of Olympic speed skaters, the **slideboard** consists of a slick sliding surface with bumpers on each end. Special nylon booties enable you to slide back and forth across the length of the board. Depending on the exercises you choose, the slideboard can be used for both aerobic and anaerobic training—and provides other athletic benefits as well, as we'll see below.

BENEFITS OF LATERAL TRAINING

Most sports that require cardiovascular fitness also require a great deal of lateral, or side-to-side, movement. Unfortunately, most traditional aerobic training machines—treadmills, stationary bicycles, stair steppers, and so on—impose little or no lateral stress, and therefore do not effectively develop your functional sports ability.

The slideboard is an exception, providing both aerobic and functional sports benefits. The side-to-side motion of sliding requires muscular contractions in combinations that closely emulate sports activities. The balancing act of stabilization enhances body awareness and fine motor skills, improving timing and coordination. In general, sliding strengthens tendons and ligaments, increases cardiovascular and muscular endurance, and improves lateral agility and power—all critical requirements for most athletic activities. Finally, because it is a low-impact activity, slideboarding is an excellent choice for both general conditioning and weight loss.

Sports and Activities Supported by Slideboarding

■ General fitness

■ Weight loss

■ Basketball

■ Tennis/Racquetball

■ Football

■ Baseball

■ Martial arts

■ Volleyball

■ Ice/In-line skating

■ Cross-country skiing

CHOOSING A SLIDEBOARD

The typical slideboard is 2 feet wide and 6 to 10 feet long. Both **rigid** (permanent) and **flexible** (portable) models are available—each has advantages and disadvantages.

Rigid Boards

Rigid boards provide a slicker, more consistent surface, are adjustable in length and work better for power training. But they're also expensive and cumbersome, and they require waxing.

Flexible Boards

Flexible boards are portable (weighing just 8 to 12 lbs), less expensive, and easily stored in a closet. Even when waxed, they have a slower surface than rigid boards. They're non-adjustable and tend to slip along the ground when you're doing high-speed power training.

The portable model will suit almost everyone's needs. But if money is no object, the rigid boards are more fun.

THE EXERCISES

The Learning Stroke

It takes only a few minutes of practice to develop the basic balance required for using a slideboard. Begin by making sure the surrounding area is clear of anything you might run into in the event of a spill, because you may slide off the board a few times during the learning stage. Then lightly run a foot over the surface of the board with your booties on to get a feel for its degree of slickness.

Starting Position

Stand on one end of the board with the side of one foot against the bumper (Fig. 10a). Place your hands on your thighs and bend slightly at the hip and knees. If possible, practice in front of a large mirror so you can watch your form.

Execution

Each slide stroke has three distinct phases—the *push*, the *glide*, and the *regroup*.

With your weight on your outer foot, *push* off across the surface. Start slowly to determine the amount of force required.

Don't worry if you don't reach the other side on your first few attempts; push a little harder each time until you get the hang of it.

After each push, *glide* with your legs in a partial split position and your weight centered between them (Fig. 10b). If you don't reach the other bumper, just keep your feet wide until you come to a stop, move over to the bumper and try again. Don't push off from the middle of the board or try to propel yourself by shuffling your feet (see Fig. 11—Wrong!). Resist the tendency to pull your feet together during the glide phase—this could lead to a fall and possible injury. At the same time, don't overemphasize the split. Simply keep your weight distributed evenly on both feet.

As you reach the opposite side of the board, *regroup* by contacting the bumper with the side of the foot (not the toe), bringing your feet together, and then pushing off again (Fig. 10c).

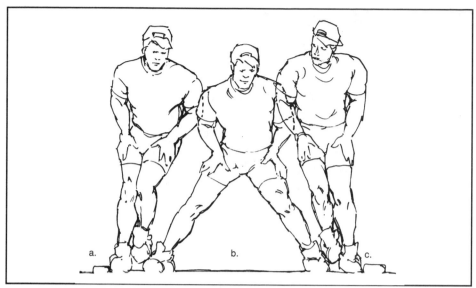

Fig. 10 — The Learning Stroke

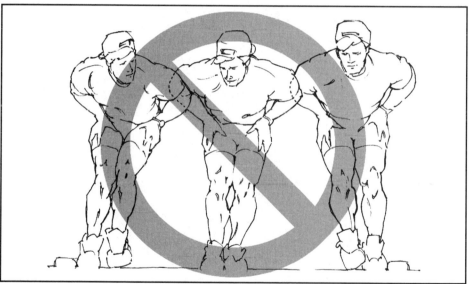

Fig. 11 — WRONG! Don't shuffle your feet or try ot push off from the center of the board.

After about 20 minutes of practicing the Learning Stroke, you will be ready to move on to the basic slide movement. This involves the same elements as the Learning Stroke, melded together in a fluid, rhythmic movement.

Basic Stroke

Starting Position

Stand on one end of the board with feet together and the side of one foot against the bumper. With your hands on your thighs, bend deeper at the knees and hips—anywhere from 50 to 90 degrees at the knee (Fig. 12a). The deeper you bend, the more you will feel the movement in your glutes and lower back. In the beginning, use your arms to support some of the weight of your upper body and to reduce the pressure on the lower back. After several weeks or more of practice, you can move on to the more advanced versions of the exercise.

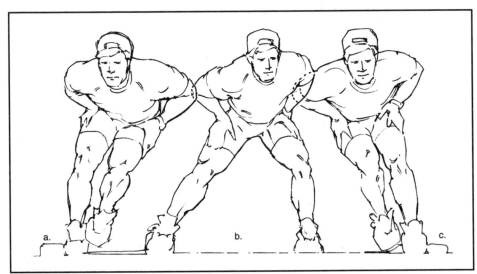

Fig. 12 — The Basic Stroke

Execution

Like the Learning Stroke, the Basic Stroke has three distinct phases—*push*, *glide*, and *regroup*.

The *push* starts in the glutes, is transmitted through the thigh, knee, and calf, and ends with a thrust of the ankle. When pushing, try to keep the force on the side of the heel—not the toe (Fig. 13). Also, keep your body facing forward and avoid turning toward the bumper.

As you *glide*, shift your weight to the inside (leading) foot (Fig. 12b). Notice how the push-leg drags behind; don't pull it in until you hit the bumper.

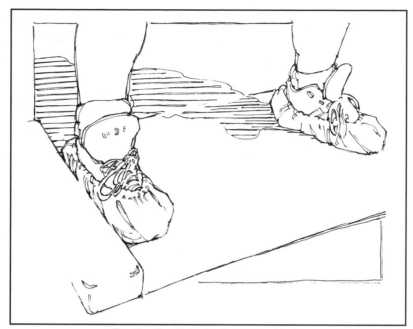

Fig. 13 — Detail: Push off with side of foot.

Contact the bumper with the side of the foot (toward the heel, not the toe) and *regroup* by bringing your feet together, and then pushing back to the other side (Fig. 12c).

Maintain a level torso as you slide and avoid bobbing or twisting as you go from phase to phase (see Fig. 14—wrong!).

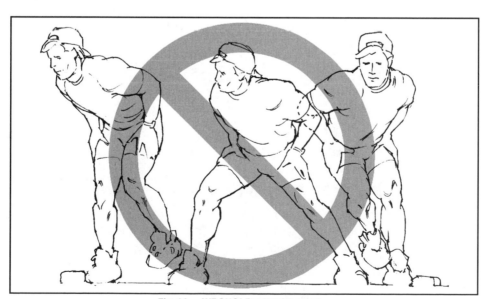

Fig. 14 — WRONG! Don't twist or bob.

You can increase the level of difficulty of this exercise by bending deeper at the knee and hip, placing a greater stress on the glutes and lower back.

ADVANCED TECHNIQUES

Speed Skating

You can also increase the level of challenge by using traditional speed skating techniques. All three forms of speed skating use the Basic Stroke as their foundation but use different arm positions. They are described here in order of increasing difficulty. By combining them with a lowered body position, you can achieve a wide range of intensities:

❶ **Hands-Behind-Back** (Fig. 15). Placing the arms behind the back makes sliding more difficult in terms of maintaining balance and increasing cardiovascular intensity and lower back stress.

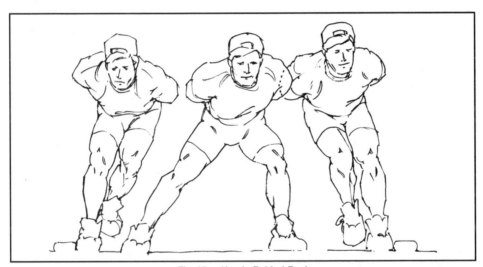

Fig. 15 — Hands-Behind-Back

❷ **Single-Arm Swing** (Fig. 16). The single-arm swing has the same merits as the first form but requires more upper body work.

❸ **Double-Arm Swing** (Fig. 17). Due to the substantial upper-body work of this technique, it is significantly more difficult than any of the other forms of sliding, and is best used for intervals and power training.

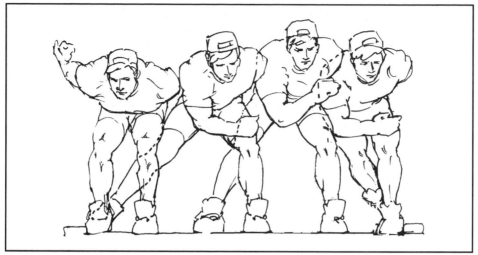

Fig. 16 — Single-Arm Swing

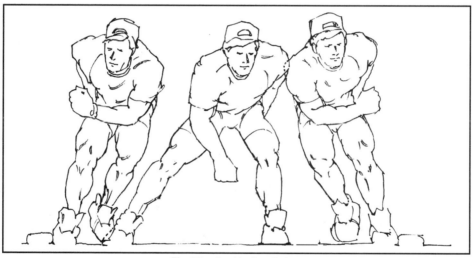

Fig. 17 — Double-Arm Swing

In addition to simulating speed skating, the slideboard can also approximate the motion of cross-country skiing. Although not as effective as a true cross-country ergometer, it provides a convenient substitute.

Cross-Country Skiing

Execution

Start by facing one of the bumpers and then, swinging your arms in opposition, shuffle your feet back and forth as though striding in place (Fig. 18). This may feel strange at first, but by visualizing the motion of cross-country skiing, you should be able to lock into the rhythm. Don't bounce, and be careful not to hit the bumper too hard with your toes.

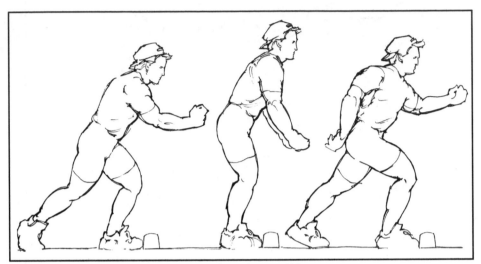

Fig. 18 — Cross-Country Skiing

THE ROUTINES

When you begin most fitness activities, it's best to start with LSD. But this just doesn't work with slideboarding! For the beginner, the intensity of even the basic sliding stroke may be difficult to maintain for long periods. Also, novice sliders sometimes experience discomfort in the legs and low back during initial periods of continuous sliding.

To give your body a chance to adapt to the stresses of using a slideboard, you need a program built on intervals, such as the Beginner Program coming up.

Don't worry if you get sore at first. Almost everyone does (especially in the glutes and inner thighs), regardless of fitness level. If your initial soreness is severe, don't slide again until you're almost back to normal. Soreness is your body's way of saying *I'm not recovered yet*, and remember, for the most part, it's the *recovery* from working out—not the workout itself—that improves your fitness level. So listen to your body and take your time working through the different programs.

Frequency

■ 3 to 4 days per week

Intensity

■ Below lactate threshold, if possible

■ Using the basic stroke, maintain a slow-to-moderate cadence. Keep in mind that sliding is very intense for new participants and that your heart rate may tend toward the upper end of the intensity range (at or above your lactate threshold). It's a good idea to monitor your heart rate at the end of each interval (or better yet, use a heart-rate monitor). If your heart rate becomes too high, or if the workout just feels too difficult, slow to a more comfortable pace. Regardless of pace, though, be sure to maintain proper form!

Time

■ For the first few workouts, perform 5 to 10 intervals in the following manner: One minute of on-time (work) followed by one minute of off-time (rest).

Progression

■ At each successive workout, add 1 to 2 intervals. Don't progress to the specific routines until you can complete at least 10 total intervals (20 minutes total: 10 minutes on, 10 minutes off).

Beginner Program

For weight loss, your exact routine will depend on many factors, including current fitness level, age, and amount of excess bodyfat. Use the following routines as a starting point. If you find the lower levels are too easy, skip ahead to a more difficult level. You should have a good idea of where you belong on this progression after a week or two.

Weight-Loss Training

To maintain as much muscle mass as possible while losing excess fat, you have to keep training intensity for prolonged sessions low. Follow the weight loss routine described below but keep your heart rate 10 to 15 b.p.m. below your lactate threshold heart rate. We highly recommend a heart-rate monitor for all bodybuilders doing aerobic work!

Fat Loss for Bodybuilders

Frequency

■ These weight-loss routines should be performed 3 to 6 days per week, 1 to 3 times per day. Start by doing Level 1 three days per week, and work up to 6 or 7 days per week before moving on to Level 2. Your sense of fatigue may rise as you increase the number of training days. If so, don't be afraid to cut back to fewer days until you feel ready to handle more. Always progress at your own pace!

Intensity

■ **For LSD:** Below lactate threshold, if possible

■ **For High-Intensity Intervals:** Above lactate threshold

■ Remember, the goal is to maximize caloric impact, not intensity.

Time

Caution: Do not attempt these routines until you have completed the Beginners Program!

■ Levels 2 through 9 all involve 30 minutes of total sliding time with progressively longer working intervals, and progressively fewer rest intervals.

■ **Level 1** — start with 5 sets of 2 minutes on and 2 minutes off. (10 minutes of slide time) Work up to 15 sets (30 minutes of slide time), before moving on to Level 2

■ **Level 2** — 6 sets of 5 minutes on, 3 minutes off

■ **Level 3** — 3 sets of 8 minutes on and 4 minutes off, followed by one set of 6 minutes on

■ **Level 4** — 3 sets of 10 minutes on and 5 minutes off

■ **Level 5** — 2 sets of 12 on and 6 minutes off, followed by 1 set of 6 minutes on

■ **Level 6** — 2 sets of 15 minutes on and 7 minutes off

■ **Level 7** — 1 set of 20 minutes on and 7 minutes off, followed by 1 set of 10 minutes on

■ **Level 8** — 1 set of 25 minutes on and 7 minutes off, followed by 1 set of 5 minutes on

■ **Level 9** — 1 set of 30 minutes on

Progression

■ Once you can slide continuously for 30 minutes, begin adding 3 minutes to your workout every 1 to 2 weeks. Caution: If you start to develop any signs of overuse injuries to the feet, ankles, knees or low back, cut back on your per-session slide time or on your total number of slides per week.

CALCULATING CALORIC EXPENDITURE FROM SLIDEBOARDING

Use the following formula to calculate approximate energy expenditure during slideboarding:

calories per minute = body weight (in pounds)   x .0945
or body weight (in kilograms) x .208

Example: Take a 175 lb. person who slides for 20 minutes of actual slide time (don't count rest intervals)

175 lbs. x .0945 = 16.5 calories per minute
16.5 calories x 20 minutes = 330 total calories

Maximum Endurance

Since there are no slideboard competitions, full-blown training aimed specifically at building sliding endurance is inappropriate. Slideboards are sometimes used by ice- or in-line skaters when they cannot get on-blade time. But then slideboard training is merely a small part of the skater's training regimen and is used to improve skating—not sliding.

General Fitness

For general fitness and cardiovascular health, LSD training is all you need. LSD training improves VO_2 max, decreasing the risk of heart disease and promoting general good health.

Although lactate threshold training isn't necessary to achieve general fitness, you may want to do some anyway. It poses a greater challenge than LSD, relieves boredom, improves lactate tolerance, and increases the rate of improvement in cardiovascular fitness. If you decide to try some threshold training, work through the LSD program first.

LSD
(VO$_2$ Max)
Training

Frequency

■ 3 to 6 days per week

■ All of the following routines are meant to be performed 3 to 6 days per week, 1 to 3 times per day. Begin with one workout per day on Level 1, three days per week. Work through all seven levels before increasing the frequency or intensity of training.

Intensity

■ Below lactate threshold, if possible

■ Keep your intensity below the lactate threshold (see Chapter 10 for further information).

■ Note: The intervals in this routine are of low to moderate intensity. They are intended for increasing VO$_2$ max and getting used to the slideboard, not for lactate threshold training.

Time

■ *Caution: Do not attempt these routines until you have completed the Beginners Program!*

■ The exact routine an individual should follow will depend on many factors, including current fitness level, age, and amount of excess bodyfat. Use the following routines as a starting point: If you find the lower levels to be too easy, skip ahead to a more difficult level. After a week or two, you should have a good idea of where you belong on this progression.

■ Levels 2 through 7 all involve 20 minutes of total sliding time with progressively longer working intervals and progressively fewer rest intervals.

■ **Level 1** — Start with 5 sets of 2 minutes on, 2 minutes off (10 minutes of slide time). Work up to 10 sets (20 minutes) before moving on to Level 2

■ **Level 2** — 4 sets of 5 minutes on, 3 minutes off

■ **Level 3** — 2 sets of 8 minutes on, 4 minutes off, followed by one set of 4 minutes on

■ **Level 4** — 2 sets of 10 minutes on, 5 minutes off

■ **Level 5** — 1 set of 12 on and 6 minutes off, followed by 1 set of 8 minutes on

- **Level 6** — 1 set of 15 minutes on and 7 minutes off, followed by 1 set of 5 minutes on
- **Level 7** — 1 set of 20 minutes

Progression

- Once you can slide continuously for 20 minutes, start adding 2 to 3 minutes to your slide time every 1 to 2 weeks. To further increase the workload, add more weekly sessions (up to 2 to 3 workouts per day and 6 to 7 days per week) or increase the workout intensity. **Caution: If you start to develop any signs of overuse injuries to the feet, ankles, knees or low back, cut back on your per-session slide time or on the total number of slides per week.**

Caution: Due to its high intensity and potential to cause injury, do not use this routine until you have completed Level 7 of the VO2 max routine above!

Frequency

- 1 to 2 times per week

Intensity

- Above lactate threshold but below VO2 max. Use the Talk Test to determine whether you are working above the lactate threshold—if so, you should be unable to maintain a conversation during the work interval. But keep in mind that this is not full-speed training; maintain a fast pace but don't go full-out.

Time

- Perform work intervals of 3 to 5 minutes, adding up to 10 to 20 minutes of total on-time. Use a work-to-rest ratio of 2-to-1 (for example, 3 minutes on-time followed by 1.5 minutes off-time).
- **Level 1** — 3 sets of 3 minutes on, 1.5 minutes off
- **Level 2** — 4 sets of 3 minutes on, 1.5 minutes off
- **Level 3** — 5 sets of 3 minutes on, 1.5 minutes off
- **Level 4** — 6 sets of 3 minutes on, 1.5 minutes off

Lactate Threshold Training

Progression

■ Keeping the above guideline in mind, adjust the total number of intervals to meet your personal needs and do no more than 20 minutes of total on-time twice per week.

Power Training on the Slideboard

High-intensity sliding is an excellent way to enhance the lateral movement power of the body. For power training, use the deeply bent knee position, along with the double-arm swing technique (see page 118). *Caution: Portable boards are prone to slipping during high-speed power training. Be careful!*

Frequency

■ 2 to 3 times per week.

■ When used for power training, slideboarding should be treated like any other form of high-intensity resistance work and done during your weight-training routine for the legs (e.g., after squats).

Intensity

■ Maximum speed.

■ To maintain maximum speed through every set, count the total number strokes that can be completed per set and strive to keep that number constant.

Time

■ 3 to 5 sets of 30 to 60 seconds each, with 2 to 4 minutes of rest between sets.

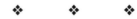

15

JUMPING ROPE

As an aerobic exercise, jumping rope has a lot to recommend it. It requires minimal equipment and space, works moderately well for VO$_2$ max and extremely well for lactate threshold work—and it's fun! Also, no other type of training will strengthen your calves as efficiently as rope jumping, making it the ideal supplementary exercise for any sport requiring fast footwork.

Let's start our exploration of rope jumping by looking at the one piece of equipment you need to get started. Then, we'll cover the exercises and lay out two basic jumping routines to bring you up to speed.

THE ROPE

You can get jump ropes of various makes and materials at most sporting goods stores. Prices range from $10 to $25; quality varies accordingly.

The cheap ones have no advantage other than price. They generally feature nylon or drapery sash cord and make for slow jumping. Even when the rope is brand-new, cheaper models often bind during jumping, due to inferior swivel pivots. The expensive ones, on the other hand, aren't that expensive and have a lot going for them. For $25 you can get a top-

TYPES OF JUMP ROPE
(In order of preference)

HANDLES		COMFORT and EASE OF USE	PRICE
	1st	Contoured wood Ball bearings	Rough-cut wood Nails or no swivels at all
	2nd	Molded plastic Ball bearings	Molded plastic Ball bearings
	3rd	Rough-cut wood Nails or no swivels at all	Contoured wood Ball bearings
ROPES		SPEED	DURABILITY
	1st	Leather	Leather
	2nd	Sash	Braided nylon
	3rd	Braided nylon	Thick plastic
	4th	Thick plastic	Sash

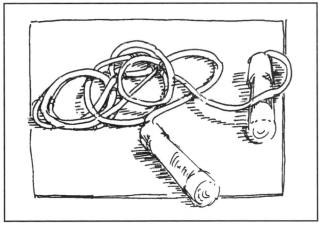

Fig.19 — A high-quality jump rope should have contoured wood handles, ball-bearing pivots, and a leather cord.

of-the-line model such as the *Everlast 4497*, with contoured wood handles, ball-bearing swivel pivots, and a fast-jumping leather cord (Fig. 19). Leather cord is more flexible than new sash and will last several years before thinning substantially at the point of ground contact.

Avoid ropes that use thick plastic cord in place of leather. These models are too slow to be useful.

ROPE LENGTH

A rope that's too short is nearly impossible to use, and one that's too long will often bounce off the ground and get tangled up in your feet. An optimum length rope will come up to about two inches above your hip bones when you stand on the center of the rope with your feet about 12 inches apart (Fig. 20).

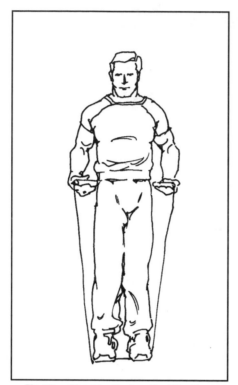

Fig. 20 — Checking the Length of the Rope

Certain types of jump ropes are adjustable—see your sporting goods retailer for assistance.

THE EXERCISES

You can jump rope in many different ways. In all cases, though, one common guideline applies: on each bounce, your feet should just barely clear the rope.

That's not as easy as it sounds, and you shouldn't be discouraged if you feel as if you're running the hurdles at first. With consistent practice, almost anyone can jump as well as a seasoned boxer.

Before you pick up your rope, practice jumping rapidly up and down, bouncing on the balls of your feet while keeping your knees *slightly* bent. Try not to let your heels touch the ground between bounces. Also, limit each bounce to a maximum of three inches. Keep your upper body as relaxed as possible throughout.

Once this feels natural, add the rope.

Start with the cord behind you and touching the tops of your heels, the handles gripped loosely, and your elbows close to your sides (Fig. 21a). Whip the rope forcefully over your head and practice your timing until you can do a long series of consecutive jumps (Fig. 21b). As your control improves, minimize each bounce until you just clear the rope and speed up the pace until you are jumping about 20 reps per 10 seconds.

The Basic Two-Footed Jump

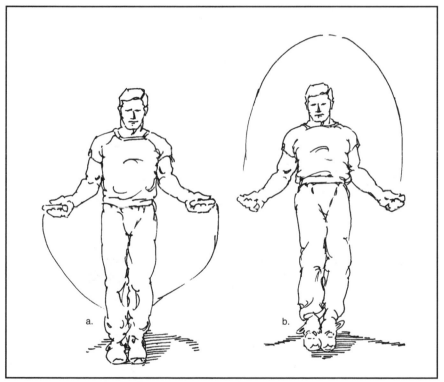

Fig. 21 — The Basic Two-Footed Jump

Side-to-Side

Imagine a line, approximately 24 inches long, running left to right under your feet. Jump with both feet together as you did in the basic movement, but bounce from one end of the line to the other (Fig. 22).

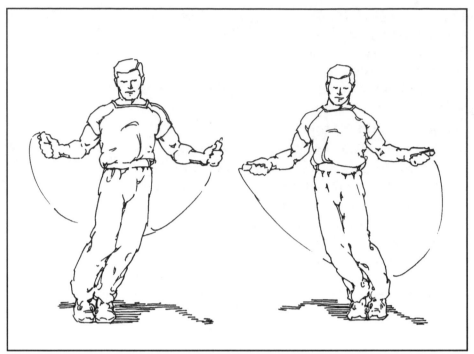

Fig. 22 — Side-to-Side

Changing Stance

This time imagine a line 24 inches long running *front to back* under your feet. Jump so that you land with one foot at each end of the line—for example, left foot forward, right foot back—and then on the next jump, reverse positions (Fig. 23).

Single-Footed Jump

This exercise places increased demands on your calves—be careful not to push it at first. Begin in the ready position. On your first jump, bend one leg at the knee and land almost straight-legged on the other foot. Bounce 5 times, then switch legs. Try alternating 5 reps right, 5 reps left without pause. In time, when your calves no longer complain about the strain, increase the number of repetitions until you can do four consecutive sets of 10 reps each leg (Fig. 24):

Execution Pattern

10 reps right, 10 reps left
10 reps right, 10 reps left
10 reps right, 10 reps left
10 reps right, 10 reps left

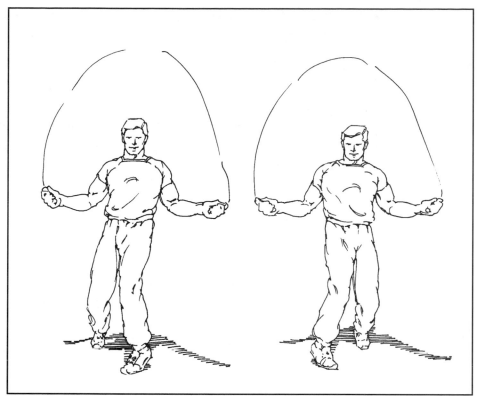

Fig. 23 — Changing Stance

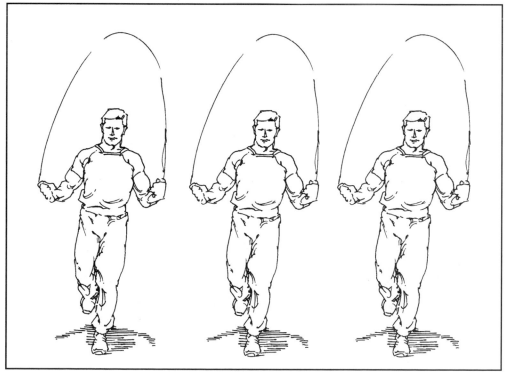

Fig. 24 — Single-Footed Jump

The next few exercises are more challenging than the previous three, and until your body learns the principle of alternate-foot jumping, you'll probably have a hard time with them. Don't get discouraged if the rope keeps catching on your rear foot. Be persistent. Chances are that when you successfully get it around once, your body will suddenly "understand" the movement and you'll soon be jumping like a pro.

Learn each exercise by working it first without your rope. Then, with the rope in hand, do the basic jump to set your rhythm and try to switch *without stopping* to the new pattern.

Single Bent-Leg Alternation

Think of this one as running in place and simultaneously jumping rope.

Begin with the basic movement. Bend your left leg back at the knee, bouncing on the ball of your right foot (Fig. 25a). Reverse legs (Fig. 25b).

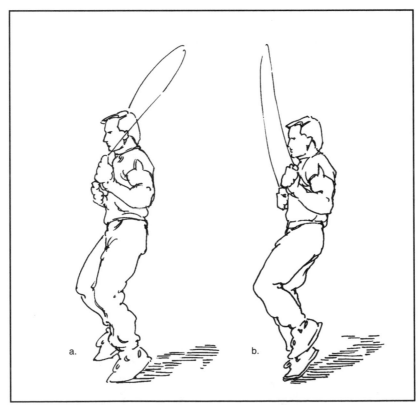

Fig. 25 — Single Bent-Leg Alternation

Straight-Leg Alternation

Begin the Basic Movement and then at some point, as you push off from the ground, extend your left leg straight forward from the hip at about 30 degrees (Fig. 26a). Bounce on the ball of your right foot. On the next bounce, reverse position: right leg extended at the hip, bounce on left foot (Fig. 26b). Repeat.

If you have trouble understanding the motion, picture the typical Russian Cossack dance done in the movies, but without the deep knee bends. Try not to let your heels touch the ground.

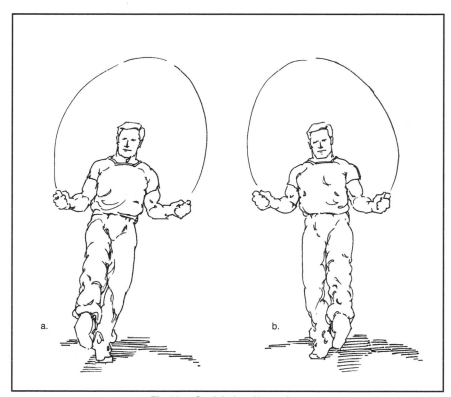

Fig. 26 — Straight-Leg Alternation

Double-Bounce Alternation

Again, begin the basic movement. At some point, as you push off from the ground, bend your left leg at the knee (Fig. 27a) and bounce on the ball of your right foot. Quickly straighten the left leg and extend it forward at the hip while you bounce for a second time on the right foot (Fig. 27b). Bring the left leg to the ground, bouncing twice on *it* as you perform the movement with your right leg (Fig. 27c,d). Continue to alternate legs.

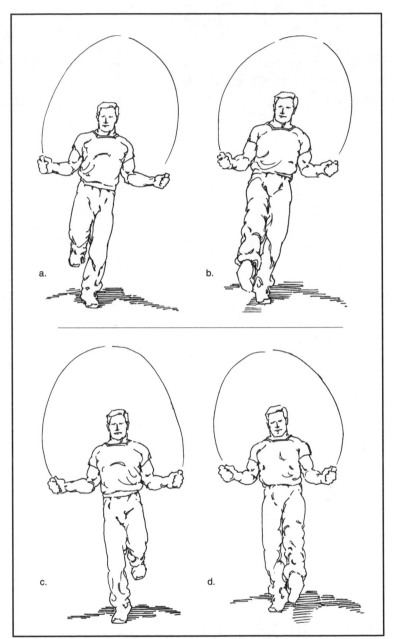

Fig. 27 — Double-Bounce Alternation

Bent-Leg Alternation

Without a rope, this would be the Mexican Hat Dance; with one, it's the Bent-Leg Alternation.

After setting your rhythm, extend your slightly bent left leg forward at the hip and then touch down your left heel after the rope has passed under. Bounce on the ball of the right foot (Fig. 28a, b).

Bring your left leg back, extend your slightly bent right leg, and touch your right heel down after the rope has passed under. Bounce on your left foot (Fig. 28c, d).

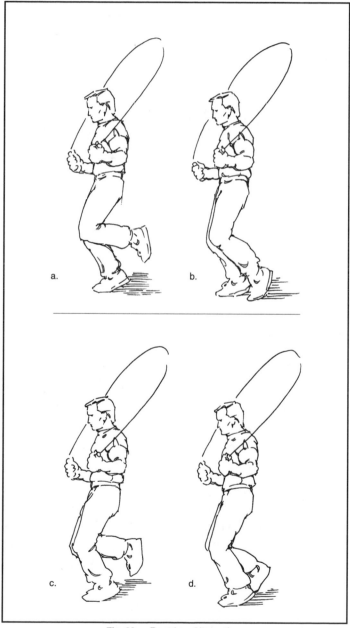

Fig. 28 — Bent-Leg Alternation

The next few exercises are trick jumps. It's best to master all the preceding moves before trying them.

Cross-Hands

Begin with the basic movement. As the rope nears the ground, cross your hands. On the next revolution, uncross them (Fig. 29).

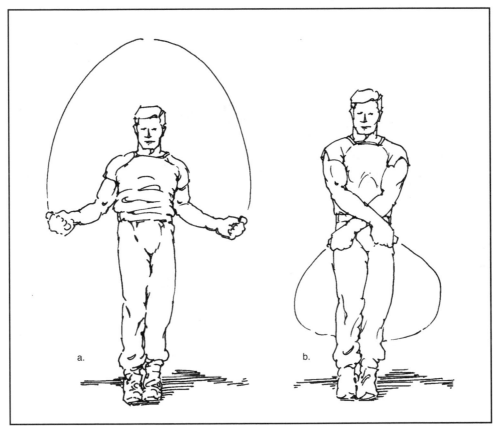

a.

b.

Fig. 29 — Cross-Hands

Figure-8

In one sense, this next exercise isn't a rope jumping move at all, because you don't jump over the rope. But it makes a great transition between other jump rope exercises (and it's flashy).

As always, begin with the basic movement. Then, as the rope passes over your head, bring both hands over to one side, as in Figure 30a. Swing the rope in a figure-8 pattern from one side of your body to the other, as shown in Figures 30b through 30f.

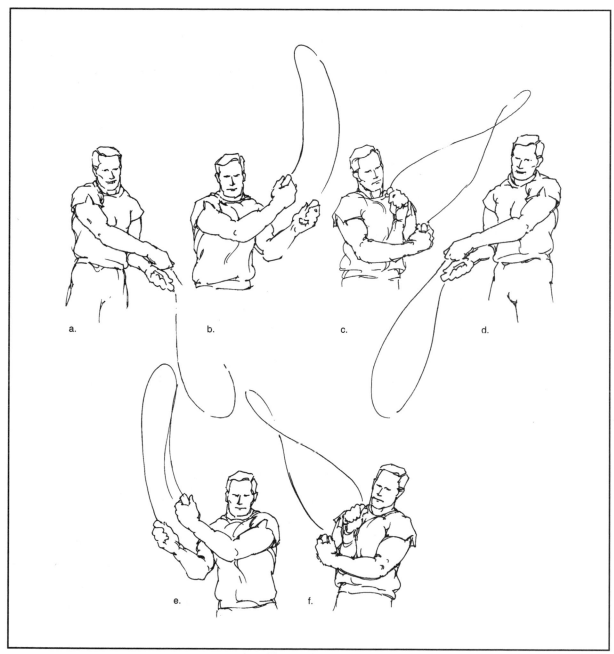

a.

b.

c.

d.

e.

f.

Fig. 30 — Figure-8

PROGRAMS

As with slideboarding, the intensity of jumping rope makes it impossible for the beginner to do LSD. Once again, you need to do intervals when you're starting out.

To minimize the danger of muscle and tendon injury, begin slowly. At first, just spend a few minutes a day working on the basic two-footed jump; when you've got it down, go through the Beginner Program below.

You should also spend some time practicing the other movements until you can bounce back and forth from one to the other easily. Aim to go for all 8 minutes (Level 3 of the General Fitness Program) without missing a step.

Beginner Program

Frequency

- 3 days per week

Intensity

- At or above lactate threshold (lower would be better but is usually impossible)
- Use the two-footed jump at a slow-to-moderate cadence. Keep in mind that jumping rope is very intense for new participants and that your heart rate may tend toward the upper end of the intensity range (e.g., well above lactate threshold). It's a good idea to monitor your heart rate at the end of each interval (or better yet, to use a heart-rate monitor during them). If your heart rate gets too high or if the workout just feels too difficult, slow to a more comfortable pace.

Time

- For the first few workouts, perform 5 to 10 intervals with as much on-time as possible up to one minute (work) followed by one minute of off-time (rest).

Progression

- At each successive workout, add 1 to 2 intervals. Don't progress to the specific routines until you can complete at least 10 total intervals (20 minutes total: 10 minutes on, 10 minutes off).

Jumping rope makes significant demands on the cardiovascular system and also on the body's ability to clear lactate. But it doesn't make the high-level demands on major muscles that running, swimming, and other intense lower-body exercises do. As a result, it's more effective for improving lactate clearance than for burning lots of calories. That makes it less than optimal as a weight-loss tool.

Training for Weight Loss or Bodybuilding Fat Loss

As we pointed out in the slideboard chapter, long steady distance (LSD) training is all you need to improve general fitness and cardiovascular health. Jumping rope is not the *best* activity for LSD because of its high impact nature, but it will work. In the interests of safety, limit individual jump rope sessions to 10 to 20 minutes.

Although jumping rope is not ideal for LSD, it's an excellent choice for interval work. Once again, it's a matter of personal preference whether to include intervals in your general-fitness program.

General Fitness

Frequency

- 3 to 6 days per week
- 1 to 2 times per day

Intensity

- The lowest possible—keep your intensity below lactate threshold, if possible

LSD (VO₂ Max) Training

Time

- *Caution: Don't try these routines until you have completed the Beginners Program!*
- As always, use the following routines as a starting point: If you find the lower levels too easy, skip ahead to a more difficult level.
- Levels 2 through 6 involve 20 minutes of total jumping time, with progressively longer working intervals and progressively fewer rest intervals.
- **Level 1** — Start with 5 sets of 2 minutes on, 2 minutes off (10 minutes of jumping time). Work up to 10 sets (20 minutes) before moving on to Level 2.

- **Level 2** — 4 sets of 5 minutes on, 3 minutes off
- **Level 3** — 2 sets of 8 minutes on, 4 minutes off, followed by one set of 4 minutes on
- **Level 4** — 2 sets of 10 minutes on, 5 minutes off
- **Level 5** — 1 set of 12 minutes on and 6 minutes off, followed by 1 set of 8 minutes on
- **Level 6** — 1 set of 15 minutes on and 7 minutes off, followed by 1 set of 5 minutes on

Progression

- Begin with one workout per day on Level 1, three days per week. Work through all seven levels before increasing the frequency or intensity of training.
- We don't recommend progressing beyond 20 minutes of on-time per session. Increase the workout intensity by jumping more quickly or using more demanding moves. *If you start to develop any signs of overuse injuries to the feet, ankles, knees or low back, cut back on your per-session jumping time or on the total number of sessions per week.*

Lactate Threshold Training

Due to the high intensity of this program and its potential to cause injury, do not use it until you have completed Level 6 of the VO$_2$ max routine above!

Frequency

- 1 to 2 times per week

Intensity

- Above lactate threshold but below VO$_2$ max.
- Use the *Talk Test* to determine whether you are working above the lactate threshold—if so, you should be unable to maintain a conversation during the work interval. But keep in mind that this is not full-speed training; maintain a fast pace but don't go full-out.

Time

- Perform work intervals of 3 to 5 minutes, adding up to 10 to 20 minutes of total on-time. Use a work-to-rest ratio of 2-to-1 (for example, 3 minutes on-time followed by 1.5 minutes off-time).

- **Level 1** — 3 sets of 3 minutes on, 1.5 minutes off
- **Level 2** — 4 sets of 3 minutes on, 1.5 minutes off
- **Level 3** — 5 sets of 3 minutes on, 1.5 minutes off

Progression

- Keeping the above guideline in mind, adjust the total number of intervals to meet your personal needs and do no more then 20 minutes of total on-time twice per week.

Overzealous jumping is often rewarded with a painful, usually long-lasting condition called **shin splints**, in which the junction between the shin bone and the calf tendons becomes inflamed. You can end up with this malady even if you don't jump on concrete or try to set endurance records your first day.

Doctors disagree about treatment. Some say rest, some say work through the pain, but our experience suggests that if the pain is slight and no tissue has been torn,* resting never seems to get you past the problem. Invariably, after a layoff, the condition reappears as soon as you start training again.

However, while jumping "through the pain" is uncomfortable, more often than not the shin splints ease off after a while and usually don't return. Consider taping your lower legs if the pain becomes too severe.

The best medicine is to proceed slowly, follow the schedule and pay close attention to the way your legs feel when you're jumping. Stop for the day at the slightest hint of pain. And in the beginning, do too little instead of too much.

❖   ❖   ❖

TRAINING ALERT: SHIN SPLINTS

*Check with your doctor if you ever have doubts concerning the extent of any injury.

PART THREE

Support

This final section covers supplementary information on aerobic conditioning necessary to train and compete at the highest level. For example, you'll read about the variety of substances athletes put into their bodies to enhance performance. The information is drawn from Health For Life's **The Human Fuel Handbook.** *The substances covered range from the vitally necessary (water) to the dangerous and much advised-against (drugs). In Chapter 19, you'll also learn how to use* **carbo-loading,** *a powerful technique for increasing endurance during long events.*

16

WATER & SPORTS DRINKS

Water is the most critical nutrient for athletic performance. Most nutrients—even essential ones—can be absent from your diet for days or even weeks without causing serious problems. But your body's water supply must be replenished frequently. This chapter explores the role of water in athletic performance and the use of sports drinks to maintain optimum fluid and electrolyte balance during prolonged exercise.

WATER—THE TEMPERATURE CONTROL SYSTEM

You are about 60% water by weight. So if you weigh 160 pounds, your body contains about 96 pounds (12 gallons) of water, only a gallon of which is in your blood.

Two-thirds of your total body water is inside your cells and is called **intracellular fluid.**

The remaining one-third is outside cells and is called **extracellular fluid.** Most of the extracellular fluid surrounds cells. Only a small part (one-twelfth of the total body water) is in blood in the form of **plasma.**

Water performs a number of vitally important functions.

First, it provides an appropriate environment for your body's many chemical reactions and for diffusion of nutrients into cells and wastes out of cells. In the form of plasma, water serves as the internal transportation system among organs, delivering nutrients and clearing wastes.

But most important to the athlete is water's function as the regulator of **body temperature.** Exercise generates heat, and this heat must be gotten rid of for exercise to continue. This is why water is critical to athletic performance—your ability to get rid of heat during exercise depends mostly on the formation and evaporation of sweat, and sweat requires water.

During prolonged exercise, you can lose a *lot* of water through sweat; if you lose enough water without replacing it, you compromise your performance: A loss of 2% of body weight through sweating causes a 10% drop in endurance and significantly impairs temperature regulation. A loss of 4% to 6% reduces both muscle endurance and muscle strength up to 30%. A loss of more than 7% may cause severe heat cramps, heat exhaustion, heat stroke, coma, and death.

Two nutrients—**sodium** and **chloride**—are lost in significant quantities through sweating. Significantly, sodium and chloride are the two elements primarily responsible for maintaining appropriate water content in the interstitial fluid (the water around the cells) and in the blood plasma.

Nutrients in Sweat

You might expect, then, that heavy sweating would lead to a deficiency of sodium and chloride in your blood plasma and interstitial fluid, and that replacing sodium and chloride would be the appropriate action. Oddly enough, just the opposite is true—**heavy sweating** *increases* the *concentrations* of sodium and chloride in your body's fluids; what you need to replace is *water*.

How can this be?

When you sweat, you lose water, sodium, and chloride, but you lose proportionately more water. The body water left behind ends up having proportionately more sodium and chloride than it did to start with. So, after sweating, the *amounts* of water, sodium, and chloride are all decreased, but the *concentration* of sodium and chloride remaining in your body is *increased*.

The amounts of sodium and chloride lost—while significant—are usually not large enough to require replacement during anything less than marathon-length exercise. Likewise, the small amounts of potassium, magnesium, and other minerals lost in sweat are not lost in quantities sufficient to require replenishment during exercise.

Fluid Intake During Exercise

Water is a different story. It is essential to drink fluids during prolonged exercise to prevent dehydration.

Dehydration causes...

- **water to be removed from inside cells** (intracellular fluid), so the chemical reactions are no longer taking place in an optimum environment
- **water to be removed from around cells** (extracellular fluid), possibly impairing diffusion of nutrients into cells and wastes away from cells
- **a drop in blood volume,** forcing the heart to pump harder and thereby increasing the stress on the heart
- **a decrease in water available for sweat,** interfering with heat dissipation and, in turn, compromising performance

Dehydration, and its negative effects on performance, are easily prevented by drinking appropriate fluids during prolonged exertion.

SPORTS DRINKS

Sports drinks are preparations that athletes drink during exercise. These are usually commercially produced. The basic goal of sports drinks is to replace water lost through sweating. Secondary goals include replacement of electrolytes lost through sweating and provision of additional energy fuel (carbohydrate, usually in the form of glucose) to spare muscle and liver glycogen stores and prolong endurance.

What to Drink

Much research has centered on determining a formulation for sports drinks that will get the water and other ingredients into your bloodstream in minimum time. Two major factors affect that time: **gastric emptying rate** and **rate of intestinal absorption**.

Gastric Emptying Rate

Gastric emptying rate refers to the speed with which the contents of the stomach empty into the small intestine, where they can be absorbed. A number of factors affect gastric emptying rate, including:

Volume. The greater the amount of stomach contents, the faster those contents enter the small intestine. This factor has little impact on the design of sports drinks. Any drink consumed in large enough quantities to bring volume-accelerated emptying into play would leave the athlete feeling bloated and most likely would interfere with sports performance.

Caloric Content. The higher the caloric content, the slower the gastric emptying rate. Caloric content seems to be the most important factor influencing gastric emptying rate. This has led some researchers to suggest that glucose and other forms of carbohydrate be left out of sports drinks because they retard emptying time. Inclusion of these substances, they hypothesize, might slow absorption of fluid enough to interfere with optimum sports performance.

However, current research indicates that under exercise conditions, plain water and an 8% (or less) carbohydrate solution exhibit similar emptying rates.

Fluid Temperature. The cooler the fluid, the faster the gastric emptying rate.

Osmolarity. This term refers to the *concentration* of particles in a given amount of fluid. For example, a cup of water with three teaspoons of sugar has a higher osmolarity than a cup of water with one teaspoon of sugar.

For many years, higher osmolarities were thought to slow gastric emptying. However, higher-osmolarity drinks are usually higher in calories as well, and researchers now believe the higher caloric values, not the difference in osmolarity, have been responsible for the slower emptying rate demonstrated in many studies.

Intestinal Absorption

The second major factor affecting the time required for the ingredients of a sports drink to get into the athlete's blood is the *rate of intestinal absorption*.

Studies show that water is absorbed much more quickly in the presence of both glucose and sodium.

In fact, although glucose slows gastric emptying, the benefits that it provides by hastening intestinal absorption and providing extra endurance fuel outweigh the drawbacks of slowed gastric emptying time. This is the basis for the first guideline

Carbodydrate Type

of what to drink during prolonged exercise: The beverage should contain some carbohydrate.

Many studies demonstrate that consuming carbohydrate during exercise effectively increases endurance. The best type of carbohydrate to include in sports drinks remains controversial.

Glucose polymers. Glucose polymers are long chains of glucose molecules, or *polysaccharides*. Since the glucose molecules in glucose polymers are all tied up in long glucose polymer chains, the osmolarity (particle concentration) of a glucose-polymer drink is low, even though the calorie content is high. This has led some manufacturers to use glucose polymers in their sports drinks, based on the thinking that the lower osmolarity will increase the gastric emptying rate, improving the efficacy of the drink.

Research shows this is not the case. Ingestion of a glucose polymer solution during exercise results in similar times for gastric emptying and intestinal absorption as the ingestion of an equal-calorie, equal-volume glucose solution. This means that glucose polymer solutions are no more effective than straight glucose solutions at getting fluid into your bloodstream quickly.

Fructose. Fructose stimulates slightly less intestinal water absorption than the same concentration glucose solution and thus is slightly less effective at getting the fluid into your bloodstream quickly. Also, high-concentration fructose solutions (greater than 2%) have been shown to cause gastrointestinal distress and diarrhea, both during rest and exercise.

On the other hand—low-concentration fructose solutions (below 2%), do not cause gastrointestinal distress, and appear to increase resynthesis of glycogen in the liver during exercise lasting over 4 hours. This resynthesis improves endurance in prolonged events such as a marathon or ultra-marathon, making small amounts of fructose an appropriate addition to sports drinks.

Sucrose. Sucrose is rapidly broken down in the small intestine to glucose and fructose. The fructose portion is associated with slightly less water absorption, as indicated above. So sucrose is a slightly less effective carbohydrate to include in sports drinks than glucose.

The second guideline: The best carbohydrate to include in a sports drink are glucose, glucose polymer, sucrose, and fructose, in that order.

Sweat contains small quantities of sodium, potassium, and other minerals important for fluid balance. The loss of these minerals, called **electrolytes**, through sweating normally poses no threat to either health or performance. A post-exercise meal replenishes all electrolyte losses.

However, performance of extreme endurance events—triathlons, marathons—in the heat may necessitate some electrolyte supplementation during exercise. Electrolyte supplementation can:

- replace electrolytes lost through sweating and thus help maintain the body's electrolyte and fluid balance
- enhance glucose absorption
- prevent onset of **hyponatremia** (abnormally low blood sodium concentration) brought on by replenishing major sweat losses with water alone

Let's expand on that third point a bit. As previously explained, water losses do outweigh electrolyte losses during exercise, resulting in higher electrolyte concentrations in the blood and a greater need to replenish water than to replenish electrolytes. But it's possible to end up with *too low* a concentration of electrolytes in your blood if, during extremely prolonged exercise, you drink a really large quantity of plain water to replenish fluid losses. Using a fluid-replacement drink containing a low concentration of electrolytes will prevent this problem.

Inclusion of small amounts of electrolytes also has other benefits, including:

- increasing the absorption of water in the small intestine
- increasing the palatability of the solution, raising the likelihood that you will drink enough to meet fluid requirements of heavy exercise

Third guideline: Sports drinks for use during prolonged endurance exercise should contain low concentrations of electrolytes, including sodium, potassium, and chloride.

Electrolyte Content

What to Drink:
The Bottom Line

For exercise up to 1 hour, the only real requirement is water. Over 1 hour, your sports drink should include low concentrations of electrolytes.

Also, for any continuous exercise over 1 hour, drinking a sports drink that contains carbohydrate (preferably glucose, glucose polymer, or sucrose) may increase your endurance.

How Much to Drink

We pointed out that large volumes of fluid—a pint or more—empty faster from the stomach than smaller amounts. However, such large amounts are impractical to drink during athletic competition. They can make you feel bloated and may interfere with optimum performance.

A better amount seems to be about 150 to 250 milliliters (roughly six ounces).

How Often to Drink

You should drink about six ounces every 10 to 15 minutes during prolonged exercise (anything over half an hour). Don't rely on thirst to tell you how much to drink. Thirst is a poor indicator of fluid needs—if you rely on thirst, you won't drink enough.

A Final Caution:
Salt Tablets

It used to be common for athletes to take salt tablets when exercising in hot weather. The belief was that since salt was lost in sweat, it should be replaced to keep the body's water and electrolytes in balance. This belief contains a grain of truth, at least for prolonged endurance exercise (as explained above), but using salt tablets to replenish electrolyte losses is not the right solution.

A *low*-concentration solution of sodium and other electrolytes, such as is found in most commercial sports drinks, is the best way to address electrolyte losses. The high concentration of sodium and chloride from salt tablets is dangerous overkill that increases the load on your kidneys, can cause nausea and vomiting, and can accelerate dehydration. Stay away from these!

Here's a summary of the guidelines covered in this chapter:

■ Don't rely on thirst to tell you when and how much to drink. Thirst is a poor indicator of fluid needs.

■ For events over one half hour, drink approximately 6 ounces of water (or sports beverage) every 10 to 15 minutes.

■ For events up to 1 hour long, water is an adequate replenishment drink. For events over 1 hour, a sports beverage is preferable.

■ A sports drink containing up to an 8% concentration of carbohydrate (preferably as glucose, glucose polymer, or sucrose) will increase endurance without slowing gastric emptying time.

■ Don't take salt tablets! They exacerbate the problem of increased sodium and chloride concentrations caused by sweating, put a strain on your kidneys, may cause nausea and vomiting, and can accelerate dehydration.

❖　　❖　　❖

GUIDELINES FOR WATER REPLENISHMENT DURING EXERCISE

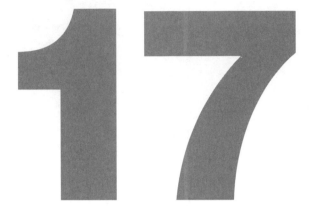

DRUGS

If you're a serious athlete, you will undoubtedly be exposed to drugs at some point and perhaps will be tempted to give them a try. The purpose of this chapter is not to moralize, but rather to discuss what drugs athletes take to enhance aerobic performance and what the drugs' effects are.

It is easy to understand why drug use among athletes is so common. Athletes—especially serious competitive athletes—operate under intense pressure. Because the smallest advantage can make the difference between winning and losing, athletes frequently believe they have no choice but to take drugs if they are to remain competitive.

Unfortunately, this perception is sometimes correct. The defensive lineman playing under an amphetamine-induced "rage" may indeed be more effective than his drug-free counterpart. The sprinter or hurdler using anabolic steroids may in fact be able to set higher records than would be possible without the use of drugs.

The question in such instances is not whether drugs give the athlete the competitive edge—it's whether having the competitive edge is worth taking the drugs.

Although the controversy over drug use in sports has grown dramatically in recent years, the practice is not new. Athletes as far back as ancient Greece, Rome, and Egypt used various potions and substances to enhance performance. For more than 2000 years, athletes have attempted to augment their physical capabilities by following special diets or ingesting particular substances.

Only relatively recently, however, as chemical technology has become more sophisticated, has drug use become widespread. In the late 1800s, competitive cyclists were the best-known drug users. The grueling six-day bicycle races of that period placed extreme physical and psychological demands on these athletes, and many turned to stimulants of one sort or another for support.

Caffeine, cocaine, heroin, and even strychnine were among the substances frequently used. The same substances were often used by boxers in this period.

In the early years of the twentieth century, money and gambling began to play bigger roles in boxing and other sports. As the financial stakes grew larger, so did the incentive to boost performance with drugs. Since many drugs were available over the counter and no testing was done, the use of drugs—especially among professional athletes—continued uncontrolled throughout the early part of the century.

Amphetamine-like stimulants, introduced in the 1930s, offered athletes a new world of performance enhancement. These stimulants were developed extensively during World War II, and were given to the troops to keep them alert and delay fatigue. After the war, stimulant use in sports dramatically increased as the soldiers came home and the prize money continued to grow.

It was not until the 1960s however, that the current controversy over drug use really began.

At the 1960 Olympics, 23 year old Danish cyclist Knud Jensen died during time trials after taking amphetamines. In 1967, Tommy Simpson, a 29 year old world-class cyclist, died during the Tour de France, also after taking amphetamines. In 1968, the International Olympic Committee began random drug testing at the Olympic games in Grenoble and Mexico City.

Over the next 10 years, many athletes were disqualified from important competitions because of positive tests for amphetamines. Eight weight lifters were disqualified from the 1970 World Weightlifting Championships; seven athletes were dis-

ATHLETIC DRUG USE: A HISTORICAL PERSPECTIVE

qualified from the 1972 Munich Olympic Games; a distance runner was disqualified from the 1975 Pan-American Games; a cross-country skier lost a bronze medal at the 1976 Innsbruck Olympic Games; a 100-meter runner lost a gold medal at the 1988 Olympic Games.

Many officials believed the program of random drug testing was bringing the problem under control, but they were wrong. What was actually happening was that athletes were simply switching to drugs that were either not yet on the banned list or not yet detectable by testing. Most prevalent among those alternative drugs during this period were anabolic steroids.

Although the International Amateur Athletics Federation and the U.S. Amateur Athletic Union banned anabolic steroids in 1970 and 1971 respectively, it was not until 1974 that the **radioimmunoassay** method of steroid testing was shown to be effective.

The International Olympic Committee quickly added anabolic steroids to their rapidly increasing list of banned drugs, and eight athletes—seven of whom were weight lifters—were disqualified for steroid use at the 1976 Olympic games in Montreal. In the following years, a large number of athletes from many different countries were disqualified from competitions on the basis of steroid use.

In the past few years, cocaine has surfaced as a prevalent drug among athletes. A number of major league baseball players have sought treatment for cocaine abuse. The most tragic case was that of college basketball star Len Bias, who died from cocaine use within hours of being drafted by the Boston Celtics.

All of these events have contributed to the present widespread public concern about drug use by athletes. With this background in mind, let's take a look at the various drugs and see:

- whether they do or do not enhance performance
- what side effects they might have
- what the long-term effects of their use might be

STIMULANTS

Athletes generally use stimulants in hopes of increasing alertness, prolonging exercise endurance, and delaying the onset of fatigue. Stimulants have been most popular in sports where aerobic endurance is critical, such as cycling and soccer. Additionally, some stimulants produce a "rage" response, which has made them popular among athletes in sports such as football, where increased aggression is valued.

Not all stimulants are alike, of course, and their status in law and sport varies considerably. Some—such as amphetamines—are illegal in most countries. Others—such as caffeine—are legal and freely available. To understand the basic differences among stimulants, let's consider the ways the various drugs achieve their physiological and psychological effects.

Sympathomimetic Amines

Your body reacts to stress through its **sympathetic nervous system**—the system responsible for the **fight-or-flight** response. That system, in response to stress, releases several hormones (adrenaline, noradrenaline, and corticosteroids) which, together, result in increased heart output, more blood to your muscles, and higher blood sugar levels. These effects ensure that your muscles receive a steady supply of oxygen and nutrients, and that waste products are efficiently removed.

Certain drugs mimic these actions of adrenaline and noradrenaline. Such drugs are called, appropriately enough, **sympathomimetic amines**, because they are *mimetic* of—that is, they mimic—the actions of these compounds released by the sympathetic nervous system.

Many of these can be purchased over the counter. The family of sympathomimetic amines includes *chlorprenaline, ephedrine* (found in Bronkaid tablets, Nyquil, and several hemorrhoidal preparations), *etafedrine, isoetharine, isoprenaline, methoxyphenamine, methylephedrine*, and similar compounds—all of which have been banned by the International Olympic Committee.

There is little evidence that any of the drugs in this group actually improve athletic performance, and only a few athletes have ever been disqualified for having used them.

Problems in this area usually occur because certain nasal sprays and asthma medications contains sympathomimetic amines as their active ingredients. Athletes using these medications should consult their doctors to avoid unexpected problems and should be aware that derivatives of the substance *imidazoline*—which does not stimulate the central nervous system—*are* permitted for use as nasal decongestants.

Potential side effects of sympathomimetic amines—at higher than therapeutic doses—include increased blood pressure, nausea, dizziness, and insomnia.

Psychomotor Stimulants

Psychomotor stimulants have roughly the same effect on the sympathetic nervous system as the sympathomimetic amines we just discussed. However, in addition, these drugs affect the *brain*, resulting in a strong feeling of confidence and well-being. As a result, these drugs are very popular among athletes.

Psychomotor stimulants—all of which are banned by the International Olympic Committee—include *amphetamines, benzphetamine, cocaine, dimethylamphetamine, methylamphetamine, norpseudoephedrine, pemoline, phendimetrazine, pipradol, preolintane,* and a large number of other related compounds. Anything thought of as "speed" is almost certainly included in this group.

The psychomotor stimulants influence the athlete's behavior and mood by affecting the activity of **neurotransmitters** in the brain.

Neurotransmitters are chemical compounds that carry messages between the brain cells. Certain neurotransmitters—such as noradrenaline and dopamine—are linked to behavior and mood. Some psychomotor stimulants, such as amphetamines, actually *increase* the production and release of dopamine and noradrenaline, and thereby elevate the athlete's mood. In addition, amphetamines increase the flow of neurotransmitters in the part of the brain that initiates body movement, lowering the threshold for motor activity.

Does all this mean that amphetamines can improve athletic performance?

The answer appears to be *yes, to a significant degree.* They definitely do not improve athletic *skill.* But, according to the results of some studies, amphetamines appear to prolong *endurance* by perhaps 3% to 5%.

That amount can be pivotal, all other things being equal, among athletes at the highest levels of competition. For this reason, this gain is sometimes referred to as the **amphetamine margin.**

The risks to be weighed against this small gain are many and serious—especially when higher doses are taken.

Psychomotor stimulants can affect the cardiovascular system, causing heart palpitations and high blood pressure. They can affect the gastrointestinal system, causing constipation or diarrhea. They can also affect the hormonal system, causing a loss of sex drive and even impotence. During athletic performance, they can mask the physiological signals of overexertion. It was this effect that caused Tommy Simpson to die of heat exhaustion during the 1967 Tour de France.

In addition, psychomotor stimulants are highly addictive. The body quickly develops a tolerance to them and needs larger doses to achieve the same effects. Withdrawal produces severe depression, so the athlete taking them becomes unable to perform without them.

The other disturbing aspect of psychomotor stimulants is that their beneficial effects are not reliable.

These drugs sometimes hinder rather than help athletic performance. Potential negative effects include impaired judgment, insomnia, headaches, and feelings of apathy and depression.

At the extreme negative end of the scale is something called **amphetamine psychosis**—a drug-induced state that closely resembles paranoid schizophrenia. In this condition—which is brought on by large doses of amphetamines—the athlete suffers from hallucinations and feelings of persecution, and may behave irrationally or even aggressively (this is the source of the amphetamine rage referred to above).

Fortunately, the symptoms of amphetamine psychoses go away after drug use is discontinued. But as with any drug addiction, discontinuing use can be a harrowing and painful experience.

While amphetamine use among athletes appears to have declined in recent years, cocaine use has been on the rise. As the dangers become better understood, and as more well-known athletes continue to acknowledge publicly their inability to control their cocaine use, we may perhaps see a decline in that area also.

Other Central Nervous System Stimulants

The drugs in this category—with the exception of caffeine—are generally quite poisonous and very dangerous to use without close medical supervision.

Included in this group, which is also banned by the International Olympic Committee, are *amiphenazole, bemigride, caffeine, croproamide, crotethamide, doxapram, ethamivan, leptazol, nikethamide, picrotoxin, strychnine,* and a number of other related compounds.

Each of these drugs stimulates some part of the central nervous system, but in high doses can cause convulsions, followed by respiratory failure and death. Because of this risk, most of these drugs have not been widely used by athletes (although two athletes tested positive for nikethamide at the Munich Olympics).

Caffeine

The exception is caffeine.

Taken in small doses—such as the amount contained in one or two cups of coffee—caffeine seems to improve alertness and reduce fatigue or drowsiness. It also increases the heart rate and acts as a diuretic. Injected in large doses, caffeine can induce convulsions. Thus, it is important to realize that caffeine is not a totally benign substance.

A great deal of controversy exists over the effect of caffeine on endurance. The theory is that caffeine increases fat oxidation during exercise, thus *sparing* glycogen for use later in the event.

Whether caffeine actually increases endurance is uncertain—scientific studies have yielded mixed results.

Several facts can be stated about caffeine, however:

- A regular user builds up a tolerance to it. The maximum effect is achieved after withdrawal for at least four days.
- Amounts in excess of about 100 to 250 mg (one or two cups of coffee) increase tension without further increasing alertness or reducing fatigue.
- Caffeine may produce undesirable side effects, including heart palpitations, nervousness, irritability, insomnia, nausea, diarrhea, and headaches.

For a more complete discussion of caffeine, see the discussion under *Ergogenic Aids* in Chapter 18.

As drug testing becomes increasingly sophisticated, and more and more drugs become detectable through scientific methods, one might expect drug use among athletes to decrease. But instead of giving up drugs, athletes have responded by moving to different drugs—those that are as yet undetectable or are not yet banned—and by learning how to tailor their drug use to the sensitivities of the current tests.

In this section, we will discuss a few of the current practices among athletes seeking ways to gain that extra edge.

CURRENT AND FUTURE TRENDS

Eleutherococcus is an extract of a plant called *Eleutherococcus senticosus*, which grows wild in the forests of Siberia. Soviet athletes have reportedly been using eleutherococcus as a stamina-building drug for a number of years. Because it does not fall into any of the International Olympic Committee's categories of *banned* drugs, its use is legal in athletic competition.

Eleutherococcus is reportedly used widely in the former Soviet Union by individuals in stressful occupations or in occupations requiring concentration for extended periods of time. Soviet cosmonauts are said to have taken the drug during extended stays in space.

It is claimed that Eleutherococcus increases endurance, coordination, and concentration, and reduces stress. Western scientists, however, have not been able to verify these claims. A recent Swedish study looked into Eleutherococcus and concluded, "It has hitherto been impossible to find documentation confirming that [Eleutherococcus] should have a positive effect on athletic performances. The few existing reports of such an effect are not convincing."

Eleutherococcus Treatments

Although the research on *dichloracetic acid* is still in a very early phase, some scientists believe that the substance may enhance endurance by slowing the accumulation of lactic acid in the muscles during exercise.

Dichloracetic acid has produced a pronounced increase in endurance in rats, but neither the benefits nor the side effects for humans is known.

Dichloracetic Acid

Blood Doping

Red blood cell infusion, or **blood doping,** is another example of the ingenious ways in which athletes attempt to improve performance without running afoul of the drug tests.

This method involves two stages:

First, a pint or two of blood is removed from the athlete's system and then is frozen and stored. Over the next several weeks, the athlete's bone marrow, stimulated by the loss of the blood, forms more red blood cells and returns the athlete's blood volume to normal.

Then, a day or two before the competition, the stored blood is reinfused into the athlete's system, creating a *surplus* of red blood cells. With these extra red blood cells, the athlete's blood can carry more oxygen to the muscles. This could theoretically result in more efficient functioning of the muscles and increased endurance.

Research indicates that blood doping actually works. A recent study demonstrated a 15% increase in aerobic performance of middle-distance runners.

But blood doping is not without its drawbacks. If the blood used is not from the athlete but from a donor, there is the risk of transmission of hepatitis, AIDS, and other blood-borne diseases. Even if the athlete's own blood is used, the risk of infection from the reinfusion procedure is always present. In addition, the increase in the number of red blood cells also increases the viscosity (resistance to flow) of the blood, forcing the heart to work harder.

❖

None of the drugs athletes take to improve athletic performance enhance health and fitness. The best you can hope for is that the drugs will not seriously injure your health. Since so many of the drugs have negative side effects, and so many of the side effects are quite serious, we hope you will think long and hard before making drugs a part of your program.

❖　　❖　　❖

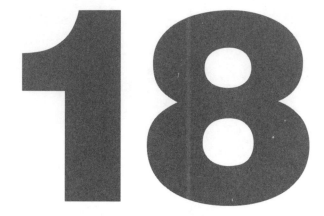

ERGOGENIC AIDS

The term **ergogenic aid** refers to any substance or process that enhances your ability to do physical work. (*Ergo* comes from the Greek word *ergon,* meaning *work; genic* means *producing.*)

Without question, the greatest ergogenic aid is **exercise.** Improvements in strength and endurance are usually quite dramatic, often exceeding 50%, in sedentary individuals who begin to exercise regularly. But when most people speak of ergogenic aids, they are usually referring to that seemingly endless variety of substances—from bee pollen to octacosanol—that athletes take to get a competitive edge.

Do any of these substances work?

THE ERGOGENIC POSSIBILITIES

There are only four ways any substance might improve your ability to produce work. These involve the way the body stores energy, utilizes energy, and translates energy into physical movement.

An ergogenic aid might:

- add to your body's energy stores, and therefore prolong endurance by increasing the amount of available fuel

■ improve your metabolism of fuel, so you use that fuel more efficiently

■ improve your endurance by slowing the accumulation of the fatigue-causing by-products of energy metabolism

■ enhance your nervous system's ability to coordinate your muscle fibers, and thereby increase your physical strength

Actually, there is a *fifth* way an ergogenic aid might work—it might make you *think* your performance will be improved. It is an established scientific fact that the mind can create physiological effects in the body based on a person's belief that a particular substance or practice will produce a certain physiological effect, even if the substance is in fact physiologically inert. This phenomenon is called the **placebo effect.** Athletes have been made to run faster, jump higher, and lift heavier weights after being given sugar pills and being told those pills were some incredible new performance drug. Likewise, doctors have cured all manner of ills, and psychiatrists have changed all manner of behaviors, using essentially empty capsules accompanied by a convincing line.

In other words, almost *anything* can improve performance if you believe it will. In this chapter, however, we'll limit our consideration to ergogenic aids that *do* have (or are at least *purported* to have) demonstrable physiological effects based on their biochemical activity, not on the placebo effect.

This chapter is not intended to be exhaustive. Far too many substances are claimed to have ergogenic qualities to explore them all here. Instead, we will focus on some of the more popular substances (many of which don't actually do anything), as well as some of the lesser known, but potentially more effective, options.

POSSIBILITY #1: MORE FUEL

Recall from Chapter 2 that your body stores energy as glycogen in your liver and muscles, and as fat in various fat deposits around your body. These energy stores are enough to see you through 2 to 3 hours of exercise, but after that, your diminishing glycogen reserves limit your endurance.

So, theoretically, one way a substance could enhance your athletic performance would be to provide extra fuel. Let's look at a few of the substances that might fall in this category.

Chemical Fuels: CP and ATP

Recall that adenosine triphosphate (ATP) and the related compound creatine phosphate (CP) are the final links in the chain of energy production. Each stores small amounts of energy in its chemical bonds and supplies the energy to make your muscles move. As soon as you start working your muscles, your ATP and CP concentrations decline dramatically. Some athletes have extrapolated from this fact that they might improve their performance by either taking ATP and CP orally or injecting them into specific muscles.

Neither method works, for two reasons:

■ First, the concentrations of these substances in the muscles fibers are not increased as by supplementation.

■ Second, even though the concentrations decline during exercise, the muscles do not become ATP-depleted; instead, the decline triggers increased carbohydrate metabolism, which keeps the muscle supplied with newly synthesized ATP.

So although it is appealing to think supplementary ATP and CP might supply extra muscle fuel, the truth is they don't.

Carbohydrates

Wait a minute—what are carbohydrates doing in a chapter on ergogenic aids? Well, remember that an ergogenic aid is something that enables you to produce more work—and right now we're looking for substances that might supply extra fuel. The number-one ergogenic in this category is carbohydrates.

As explained in the *ATP, Carbohydrate, Fat, and Protein* chapter, when you consume a diet high in complex carbohydrates, you store greater-than-usual amounts of glycogen in your muscles and liver. The stored glycogen is *fuel*, and the more of it you have, the longer you can work. So carbohydrates have a significant ergogenic potential.

This potential can be maximized, for short periods of time, through carbo-loading (to be discussed in Chapter 19). Carbo-loading enables you to store glycogen in even larger amounts than you would if you simply followed a high carbohydrate diet. These increased stores are definitely ergogenic—that is, they provide even larger amounts of fuel and so increase your ability to produce work.

Finally, carbohydrates can increase your endurance if you take them during prolonged exercise (exercise in excess of one hour). When consumed as part of a carefully prepared beverage (see Chapter 14), carbohydrates can raise your blood glucose level. Your muscles can then use this added glucose as fuel. This helps your glycogen stores last a little longer, increasing your endurance.

So ergogenic aids do not have to be exotic to work. We expect them to be because so many exotic-sounding products are marketed as ergogenic aids. But carbohydrates are a perfect illustration that informed and disciplined use of ordinary nutrients can be ergogenic.

Free Fatty Acids

Fat is an important source of energy. Your body stores much more energy as fat than as carbohydrate. The relative amounts of carbohydrates and fat you use as fuel vary constantly during different phases of exercise.

The more you burn fat, the less you have to burn glycogen; the longer the glycogen lasts, the longer you can keep going during prolonged exercise. So anything that increases the contribution fat oxidation makes to muscular energy production should increase your endurance.

Your body uses fat for energy in the form of *free fatty acids*, which circulate in your blood. This fact has led some theoreticians to speculate that endurance could be increased by finding a way to *increase* the free fatty acids in the athlete's blood.

The concept is simple: If you have more fatty acids in your blood, your muscles can use more fatty acids for energy. You therefore will use less glycogen. And you will thus have greater endurance.

Sounds logical enough.

So how do you increase the free fatty acids in your blood? Generally speaking, in only one way: with caffeine. A second way, invoking the **fight-or-flight response,** works but isn't really under voluntary control.

Caffeine, used carefully, can safely increase the level of free fatty acids in your blood, with some accompanying ergogenic effect. We will discuss caffeine in more detail in a moment.

The fight-or-flight response, what your body calls in time of danger, *naturally increases* the free fatty acids in your blood.

This happens because the fight-or-flight response causes the release of hormones called *catecholamines,* such as epinephrine (adrenaline). Catecholamines stimulate both the breakdown of fat molecules and the breakdown of glycogen, but stimulate the breakdown of fat molecules *more.*

As a result, fat oxidation increases, which may prolong glycogen stores in the long run, enhancing endurance. This may even occur to some extent as a result of normal nervousness or excitement. So when you get nervous before a big event—especially an endurance event—don't be concerned: your nervousness may mean extra energy a couple of hours down the line!

POSSIBILITY #2: BETTER METABOLISM

The amount of energy you produce, as well as the overall effect on your endurance, varies according to both the *kind* of energy-producing metabolism taking place (aerobic or anaerobic) and the particular fuel being broken down (glycogen, protein, or fat). Since these factors affect how efficiently you produce energy during exercise, it stands to reason that if you could find ways to influence those factors, you would also be able to influence energy production and endurance.

Certain ergogenics *do* promote improvements in endurance by altering metabolism. This section looks at the pluses and minuses of using these substances.

Caffeine

Caffeine is not as benign an ergogenic aid as, say, complex carbohydrates—caffeine is a drug.

What does caffeine *do* to your body? It:

- stimulates your central nervous system; this is what increases alertness and makes some people jittery
- stimulates the kidneys to produce more urine; this is what causes the well-known increase in trips to the bathroom after a cup of coffee
- increases respiratory rate
- may enhance the strength of contracting muscle

The changes are more prominent in people who do not habitually consume caffeine; in fact, many of these changes are not seen at all in habitual caffeine users.

Although study results are not unanimous, general consensus holds that caffeine improves endurance performance. It appears to accomplish this through at least three mechanisms.

First, and probably most significant, caffeine causes something similar to the fight-or-flight response—**it enhances the action of catecholamines, which in turn stimulate fat breakdown and bring about an increase in fatty acid oxidation. The net result is a relative sparing of glycogen and increased endurance.**

Second, caffeine may affect the *intensity* of exercise. In some studies, athletes taking caffeine have been found to perform at higher levels of intensity than athletes taking a placebo. How caffeine accomplishes this is not known; it may be that caffeine raises the maximum intensity level you can *tolerate* during prolonged exercise. Because tolerance is increased, your maximum effort may take you to a higher level of intensity.

Third, caffeine may influence performance through its *psychological* effects. Caffeine stimulates the central nervous system. The resulting psychological lift may cause you not to tire as quickly and to feel less muscular effort in general. Caffeine may also stimulate clear and alert thinking, which could enhance athletic performance in more subtle ways.

How much caffeine is the right amount for achieving these effects?

The best current estimate is approximately 250 to 300 milligrams*—about the amount in two cups of coffee—taken a little while before beginning prolonged exercise. See the table on the next page for the caffeine content of various sources.

If you're thinking of using caffeine as an ergogenic aid, remember that only in prolonged endurance situations is caffeine likely to help you. *Other than its potential psychological effects, none of the benefits of caffeine are available during short-term exercise.*

---

*Some new studies show significant endurance improvements on dosages as low as 100 mg.

SELECTED SOURCES
OF CAFFEINE

SOURCE	MG OF CAFFEINE (approx.)
Coffee, brewed (1 cup)	103
Black Tea (1 cup)	36
Cola (12 ounces)	46
Chocolate (1 ounce)	13

Also, because of caffeine's diuretic effect (stimulation of the kidneys), you are much more likely to become dehydrated having taken caffeine. This can seriously jeopardize performance.

Will caffeine hurt you?

In recent years investigators have disagreed strongly about caffeine's possible negative effects. But certain conclusions seem to be gaining more general acceptance.

Small amounts of caffeine—one or two cups of coffee a day—probably won't hurt you.

This is not to say a small amount of caffeine will have no effect, because it surely will. Rather, the effects at that level of intake should be more or less limited to the immediate stimulation and should not cause some of the other, more harmful effects that caffeine can cause.

Caffeine may, when taken in larger amounts, cause anxiety, heart palpitations, nervousness, irritability, insomnia, nausea, diarrhea, and headaches. Injected in large amounts, it can even cause convulsions. Caffeine may also increase risk of heart attack, cancer, and fibrocystic breast disease, but these associations remain controversial.

Caffeine is a diuretic, stimulating the kidneys to produce urine. This partially dehydrates you, and it only takes a little dehydration to limit your ability to achieve peak performance.

A regular caffeine user develops a tolerance for the drug and therefore will be less affected by taking it than someone who does not have it regularly. The maximum effect seems to be realized when the user has not had caffeine for at least four days.

Finally, ergogenic properties aside, caffeine does nothing positive for your health.

At the very best, it may improve endurance by a small amount without doing you any physical harm. However, it may cause some of the physical problems mentioned above—any one of which could hurt your athletic performance.

Psychomotor stimulants include amphetamines, cocaine, and generally anything you might think of as speed. These drugs, which produce strong feelings of confidence and well-being, have become very popular among both athletes and non-athletes (see Chapter 17.)

Psychomotor stimulants do appear to have several ergogenic effects. They:

- may increase aerobic endurance
- may decrease recovery time following work
- may work much like caffeine to increase fat oxidation and thus conserve glycogen during prolonged exercise
- may improve reaction times in athletes who are already tired
- can increase muscular strength

Against the potential benefits just listed, you have to weigh the potential harm—and the potential harm is extreme.

Physical risks include heart problems, high blood pressure, gastrointestinal disturbances, insomnia, digestive difficulties, and sexual dysfunction. Athletes have been known to die from heat exhaustion when psychomotor stimulants prevented them from recognizing their body's warnings against over-exertion.

Psychological risks include apathy, intense depression, paranoia, and psychosis.

Because psychomotor stimulants are generally very addictive, problems developing from their use may be difficult to get rid of.

Psychomotor Stimulants

POSSIBILITY #3: FEWER BY-PRODUCTS

After you reach the point during exercise—3 to 5 minutes after starting—at which oxygen reinforcements have arrived, the biggest single factor in the onset of fatigue will be your pH, or acid/base balance.

As you continue to produce lactic acid through anaerobic metabolism, your body has to work harder and harder to keep your pH balance normal. Eventually, you exceed your body's ability to buffer the lactic acid that's being produced, and you are forced to stop exercising because you feel exhausted.

Since the build-up of by-products of energy metabolism—lactic acid is the most notable of these—brings on fatigue and exhaustion, it seems logical that a substance which would slow the accumulation of those by-products might increase endurance.

This section examines a couple of substances whose ergogenic potential is based on this possibility.

Sodium Bicarbonate

One of the ways your body buffers the accumulation of lactic acid is by releasing bicarbonate. Why not beat your body to the punch, then, and take sodium bicarbonate (baking soda) orally prior to exercising?

Although the gains are small, sodium bicarbonate *does* appear to prolong endurance when taken prior to exercise. It does this by inducing *alkalosis*—a state of increased alkalinity—that in effect gives your body an **acid deficit** at the beginning of exercise. In a state of alkalosis, your body can neutralize a greater amount of acid. Since acid build-up brings on fatigue and exhaustion, neutralizing more acid slows the build-up and prolongs endurance.

Taking sodium bicarbonate appears to improve performance in short, high-intensity events, such as an 800 meter race.

In one experiment, experienced runners given 21 grams of sodium bicarbonate (the equivalent of 10.5 Alka Seltzers) over two hours prior to exercise ran an average of 2.9 seconds faster in an 800 meter race. It may not sound like much, but a 2.9 second improvement translates into a distance of 19 meters, which easily can be the difference between first and last place in an 800 meter race. Furthermore, although they didn't know if they had taken the sodium bicarbonate or a placebo, those who took the sodium bicarbonate felt they had not done well because they *had too much left at the finish line.*

Although they might not have known prior to the race whether they had gotten sodium bicarbonate or a placebo, half of them found out soon after. Approximately three hours after taking the sodium bicarbonate, the runners experienced what researchers delicately described as *urgent diarrhea*.

The long-term consequences of sports-related bicarbonate ingestion are unknown.

Water

As discussed in Chapter 16, another by-product of energy production during exercise is *heat*. This heat must be dissipated to keep your body temperature constant, so it gets transported to your skin, which is cooled by your sweat. During prolonged exercise, you can lose significant amounts of water through sweating.

Too much water loss during exercise can cause dehydration, hyperthermia (excessively high body temperature), and possibly heat stroke. These conditions may lead to severe physical problems, but well short of that they can impair athletic performance.

You can minimize water loss by replacing lost fluids during exercise. Does this make water an ergogenic aid? Yes, strictly speaking. Drinking water during prolonged heavy exercise increases your ability to keep exercising. You can also sneak in a little extra fuel by adding a small amount of sugar to your water. See Chapter 16, as well as the *During Competition* program in Chapter 19, for details on what to drink and when.

Lactic Acid

Strange as it seems, occasionally someone claims you can reduce the build-up of lactic acid during exercise by taking lactic acid *itself* as a supplement. The theory behind this claim is that the extra lactic acid will cause your muscles and liver to respond by producing more of the enzymes that help reduce lactic acid in your blood.

The problem is that you *still* have to get rid of the lactic acid as carbon dioxide and water by exhaling. The more there is to exhale, the heavier your breathing must be to keep up. So taking in more lactic acid cannot lower the amount of converted lactic acid that has to go back out.

There is no scientific research supporting the notion of taking lactic acid as an ergogenic aid.

THE ERGOGENIC GRAB BAG

This section describes some of the "ergogenic aids" for which the claims are so general (usually the claim is *increased endurance*) that it's impossible tell in which of the three groups—supplying fuel, aiding metabolism, or reducing the accumulation of by-products—the particular substance is supposed to belong.

We won't keep you in suspense—none of these substances has been shown to improve athletic performance. Nonetheless, chances are you will run into athletes who swear by them.

Octacosanol

Octacosanol is a substance that occurs naturally in wheat and other whole grains. It is present in wheat germ oil—another nutritional supplement that is unnecessary and quite expensive—and can be bought in capsule form.

Its advocates claim it improves endurance, alertness, and speed. No scientific studies have been done on octacosanol and athletic performance, so there is no evidence to support any claims made on its behalf.

Bee Pollen

The companies selling bee pollen claim it improves endurance and strength, and they usually back up these claims with endorsements from athletes who say it works for them.

Although those athletes may well believe bee pollen works for them, there is no scientific evidence to support the claims. Bee pollen contains some B vitamins and a few other nutrients, but nothing that would confer benefits beyond those available from a balanced diet.

Ginseng

Those who advocate ginseng as an ergogenic aid for athletes claim it increases resistance to stress and so raises mental and physical capacities for work. Those who advocate ginseng as a useful substance for everyone claim it slows aging, reduces hypertension, fights diabetes, cures insomnia, and prevents headaches, strokes, and various other diseases.

They also claim it is an aphrodisiac.

Ginseng use goes back thousands of years. It was written about in China as long ago as 2800 B.C. Why has it received so much attention?

One answer—a rather colorful one—comes from something called the *Doctrine of Signatures*. The Doctrine of Signatures is an ancient belief that *like cures like*—that is, that plants tell you by their physical appearance what they are good for.

For example, a plant with heart-shaped leaves would be good for the heart. A plant with red leaves would be good for the blood. And so on.

The Doctrine of Signatures sounds silly to most Westerners, but it was taken seriously for many centuries, and it helps explain why ginseng was held in such high esteem. Ancient herbalists claimed the mature root of the ginseng plant resembled a human body with four limbs. Thus, the Chinese name was *jen shen*, or *man plant*. Because the plant resembled a person, it was thought to cure all human ills.

The truth is that very little scientific research involving ginseng has been done on human beings. That may seem odd, given all the claims for ginseng, but there are two major reasons why this is so.

First, ginseng is not one uniform substance—it comes in a variety of forms. As a result, reliable preparations have been hard to come by—and scientists haven't wanted to perform experiments using unreliable preparations.

Second, reports of negative responses to ginseng are well-known, and discourage researchers from pursuing research in this area.

Some animal research has been done, and it offers some reason to think that ginseng may have some positive effects in humans. Ginseng may act as a pain killer. It may improve memory. It may reduce stress.

Unfortunately, ginseng definitely *can* have bad effects, including: diarrhea, hypertension, mastalgia (breast pain), skin eruptions, insomnia, depression, and nervousness.

There is even a recognized medical condition known as **ginseng abuse syndrome,** in which individuals become dependent on the pharmacological effects of ginseng, much as other people become dependent on caffeine. These people experience withdrawal symptoms when they stop taking ginseng.

We do know that ginseng contains a number of pharmacologically active agents, and that these agents cause ginseng's various effects. Until further research is done, using ginseng is risky—its negative effects could easily harm your performance more than its positive effects, if any, might help you.

In any event, if you experiment with ginseng, you should keep the doses small—to minimize the occurrence of the well-documented side effects.

Phosphate Loading

One product which has been marketed for years as an ergogenic is called *Stim-O-Stam*. This nutritional supplement contains mostly sodium and potassium phosphate, and is sold on the theory that replenishing phosphates lost during exercise will increase endurance and shorten recovery time. Stim-O-Stam has been widely used by college track athletes.

Muscular strength and endurance are limited by the ability to regenerate ATP (adenosine triphosphate). Although an ATP molecule *does* have three phosphates in it, ATP regeneration is not limited by the amount of phosphate present.

In fact, research indicates *phosphate loading* doesn't work. Under scientific conditions, phosphate loading does not improve endurance, recovery time, muscle power, or oxygen uptake.

Vitamin E

Since its discovery in 1923, Vitamin E (or **alpha tocopherol**, as it is called chemically) has been the subject of much speculation. Some have claimed it improves sex drive. Others have said it makes hair shine. Still others have said it improves circulation.

Several scientific studies in the 1950s seemed to indicate Vitamin E might improve athletic performance. Those early studies found Vitamin E prolonged endurance, increased utilization of oxygen, and reduced the accumulation of lactate.

But the more recent research does not support these findings. The most likely explanation for this difference is that the early research was not as well designed or as tightly controlled.

In two areas, though, Vitamin E does appear to offer some promise:

First, Vitamin E acts as an *antioxidant*, preventing certain biochemical reactions in the body that impair health and may accelerate aging.

Second, some preliminary research indicates Vitamin E may improve athletic performance at *high altitudes* (5,000 feet or more) by improving oxygen utilization. So, if you're training at high elevations, you may want to experiment with a little Vitamin E—it certainly won't hurt you.

A LAST WORD ON ERGOGENICS

As intriguing as potential ergogenics may be, they are at best a relatively small aspect of athletic nutrition. Getting caught up in the search for ergogenics can blind you to more important nutritional issues—and with that in mind, let's take a moment to describe where ergogenics fit into the overall picture.

First, remember what an ergogenic aid is. It is a process or substance that improves your ability to do work. If that is your goal, then you want to start by doing those things that will have the greatest impact on that ability. After that, you can start doing the remaining things—the ones that have less impact on your ability to do work.

The two things that have the greatest impact are regular training and good basic nutrition.

A non-exercising person who starts exercising regularly can increase his or her aerobic endurance by 50% in a short period of time. A person who eats poorly can also increase his or her endurance significantly by changing to a good balanced diet with 60% to 65% of the calories derived from complex carbohydrates. A person who does both of these at once can feel a remarkable improvement almost immediately.

So if you're not yet exercising as regularly as you should, or eating as well as you should, you're not ready to talk about ergogenic aids. It would be like putting racing tires on a car that needs a new carburetor. Get the carburetor taken care of, and *then* start thinking about those tires.

Second, remember that even those ergogenics that work don't make dramatic differences—they make *incremental* differences. Most of the benefits to be had show up at the end of a long period of exercise (like running a marathon), when you may be able to keep going for just a little bit longer than you otherwise would. So if you're not pushing yourself to the limits of your endurance, these ergogenics may have nothing to offer you.

Who, then, can benefit from ergogenic aids? A very small group of competitive athletes: those who already train regularly and seriously, follow a sound diet, get enough sleep, compete with intensity, and essentially never deviate from their training regimens—in short, those for whom tiny improvements can make the difference between winning and losing.

❖　　　❖　　　❖

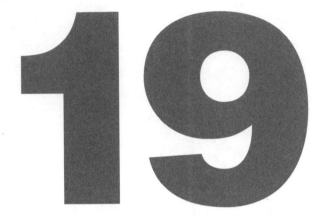

NUTRITION BEFORE, DURING & AFTER AEROBIC COMPETITION

This chapter speaks specifically to the serious aerobic athlete looking to optimize competition performance through dietary manipulation.

You should start this program 4 or 5 days prior to a competition and continue it through the day and night of the competition itself. The next day, resume your regular training diet.

This program covers three periods: the days and hours immediately *before* the competition, time *during* the competition, and the hours immediately *after* the competition.

Prior to a competition, you want to store as much glycogen as possible, to promote maximum energy and endurance when competing. *During* a competition, you want to avoid dehydration and glycogen depletion. *After* the competition, you want make sure you rehydrate adequately, so you can go on with normal training. This program is designed to accomplish all of these goals.

Details of your individual program will vary according to your sport. Glycogen storage, for example, is a more important concern if you engage in endurance competition.

Dehydration is an issue only if you compete long and hard enough to lose a lot of water through perspiration.

In short, the longer and more intense your competition, the greater the extraordinary nutritional preparation you will need.

THE *BEFORE COMPETITION* PROGRAM

The Week Before the Competition

Carbo-Loading

During the 4 or 5 days prior to competition, your goal is to build higher-than-usual glycogen stores to ensure your endurance is at its peak. This is the time for **carbo-loading.**

Carbo-loading makes use of an observed, but unexplained, physiological fact: a sudden increase in dietary carbohydrate will increase the body's storage of glycogen. The effect is even more pronounced if the increase in dietary carbohydrate is preceded by a severe depletion of body glycogen stores.

Progressively more severe versions of carbo-loading involve progressively more severe **depletes**—periods during which carbohydrate intake is restricted—prior to raising carbohydrate intake above normal. While the most severe forms of depletes do offer a slight performance benefit, this is offset by the health risks and discomfort they involve. We do not recommend the use of dietary depletes.

Some important points to keep in mind about carbo-loading:

■ Carbo-loading is only valuable if you do *endurance* exercise. Even heavy bodybuilding workouts don't come close to using up your glycogen stores. If you're not going to use up your normal reserve of glycogen, having extra glycogen won't do anything for you, because the amount of glycogen will not be the limiting factor.

■ Carbo-loading can hinder short-term, high-intensity performance. For every gram of glycogen stored in muscle, you also store 2.7 grams of water. Increase glycogen storage, you increase water storage. This can make you feel heavy and stiff during exercise.

■ Full-out carbo-loading (in its most severe form, not described here) is not a good idea. Repeated carbo-loading of this type can cause kidney and heart problems—and the long-term effects on your health are not known.

■ Athletes with diabetes or hypertriglyceridemia should check with their physician about the advisability of carbo-loading.

Below we provide two safe and effective approaches to carbo-loading:

Option One is the *diet only* approach. This method provides excellent results and is not dangerous to your health. If this approach meets your needs, use it.

Option Two is the *diet and heavy exercise* approach. This method provides even more glycogen storage and does not pose a particular threat to your health.

Determine which method fits your needs by consulting the chart below.

CARBO-LOADING SELECTION CHART

DURATION OF COMPETITION	BEST CARBO-LOADING PLAN
Less than 2 hours	No Carbo-Loading Necessary
2 to 3 hours	Option One
3 or more hours	Option Two

Option One: Diet Only

This method is very simple. For each of the 4 days immediately preceding the day of the competition, boost your intake of carbohydrates from its normal rate (probably 60 to to 65% of your calories) up to 70%. Don't begin any sooner, though—a normal training diet provides a better balance of nutrients, so you should stay on it until it's really time to start socking away glycogen for the big event.

Taper your training during those four days, and keep your calorie intake at its normal level while you raise your percentage of carbohydrate intake. For reference, the table at the top of the next page contains typical carbohydrate consumption numbers for advanced endurance athletes during regular training and carbo-loading.

TYPICAL CARBOHYDRATE CONSUMPTION
BY ENDURANCE ATHLETES

BODYWEIGHT	TRAINING DIET	CARBO-LOADING DIET
120 to 150 lbs.	400 to 600 grams	Up to 20% higher
180 to 200 lbs.	800 to 1000 grams	

Option Two: Diet and Heavy Exercise

The dietary component of this method is the same as the one explained in **Option One**. The difference here is that you add an exercise-induced glycogen depletion stage prior to starting the high-carb diet. Depleting your glycogen stores before carbo-loading allows you to store even more glycogen than you could from diet alone.

On the third or fourth day before your competition—while still on your normal training diet—exercise to exhaustion. This means having a very long, hard training session to deplete your glycogen stores as much as possible. Then for the remaining 2 to 3 days before your competition, exercise moderately to taper and follow the high-carbohydrate diet as explained under **Option One**.

This method does not pose any particular health risk and is a very effective way to prolong your endurance. Using this method, you may as much as *double* your normal glycogen reserves. And that can make a big difference when you get into the final stages of an endurance event.

SUMMARY OF CARBO-LOADING OPTIONS

OPTION	WHEN APPROPRIATE	INCLUDES
No carbo-loading	Competition less than 2 hrs. duration	Remain on **Program One**
Option 1	Competition 2 to 3 hrs. duration	4 days high-carb diet
Option 2	Competition > 3 hrs. duration	Depletion by exercise, then 2 to 3 days taper plus high-carb diet

The Day of the Competition

If you have followed one of these carbo-loading options during the week prior to competition, you will be ready to begin your event in peak nutritional condition. The final point is to make sure your body is free from discomfort at exercise time.

Avoid eating gas-producing foods, such as beans, cabbage, broccoli, and Brussels sprouts on the day of your competition. Avoid spices or anything that tends to give you indigestion. Eat very little fat. Avoid large amounts of fiber.

Eat your final pre-event meal about four hours before the starting gun. This will ensure that your digestive process will not cause you discomfort during exertion.

The meal itself should be much like the breakfasts you have been eating during the carbo-loading phase: light, very high in carbohydrates, and easy to digest. We suggest something like the following:

PRE-EVENT MEAL (about 4 hours before competition)

---

1 cup orange juice
1 cup oatmeal, no salt
2 slices whole-wheat bread with 2 tsp. jelly
1 cup tea with 2 tsp. honey

Total Calories: 454

% Calories Carbohydrates:	80	Total Sodium:	342 mg.
% Calories Protein:	11	Total Potassium:	786 mg.
% Calories Fat:	10	Total Calcium:	91 mg.
		Total Fiber:	1.5 gm.

As an alternative, you might try using a commercially prepared liquid meal as your pre-event meal. The advantage of such preparations is their rapid gastric emptying time. Because you digest them and absorb their nutrients quickly, you can have this meal as late as two hours before competition.

The disadvantage is that most of these preparations contain a higher proportion of fat and protein, and therefore a lower proportion of carbohydrates, than the solid meal suggested above.

If the liquid meals interest you, try them well in advance of competition day to see how your body responds to them. Whatever you do, don't try something brand-new on the day of a competition.

One final point: You can lose considerable fluid through sweating during competition. In preparation for taking the appropriate steps to rehydrate afterward, measure and record your bodyweight before your first heat or event.

THE *DURING COMPETITION* PROGRAM

As with carbo-loading *before* competition, the degree of nutritional support you require *during* competition depends on how long and how hard you perform. If you compete in short-duration, high-energy events such as sprinting, you probably need no nutritional support at all. If you play soccer or run long distances, some nutritional support is definitely in order.

The object of nutrition during competition is to prolong energy and endurance as long as possible. This is done by preventing you from reaching physiological barriers to continued effort. These barriers mainly relate to *fluids* and *carbohydrates*.

Fluids

Recall from our discussion of fluids in Chapter 16 that water plays a vital role in your health generally and in your athletic performance in particular. As the primary regulator of body temperature, water is the main barrier standing between you and heat stroke. Drinking fluids during prolonged exercise reduces dehydration, slows the decline in your blood plasma volume, helps delay fatigue, and improves performance. Follow these guidelines:

- Start by drinking 1 to 2 cups of water about 30 minutes before competition. This amount will carry you through short or moderate periods of exercise.

- After about 15 minutes of exercising, start drinking additional fluids—about 6 ounces every 15 to 20 minutes.

- Continue taking fluids in this manner during the entire competition—or at least during those periods in which you are actively participating. Don't wait until you're thirsty to drink—thirst is a poor and invariably late indicator of your body's needs for fluids.

■ If your competition lasts longer than 1 hour (for example, running a marathon), use a sports drink. Under 1 hour, water is sufficient. Using a sports drink containing glucose or other carbohydrate source in less than an 8% solution will increase your endurance without slowing gastric emptying.

SUMMARY OF
DURING COMPETITION
PROGRAM

TIME	ACTION
30 minutes before competition	Drink 1 or 2 cups of cold water
15 minutes into competition	Drink 6 oz. of of cold water or glucose mixture
Every 15 to 20 minutes thereafter during competition	Drink 6 oz. of of cold water or glucose mixture

THE *AFTER* COMPETITION PROGRAM

This part is not really a program as such—it is a set of concerns to keep in mind and apply to your own competitive situation. No one "program" would suffice here because of the variety of competitive conditions.

What does it mean to say *after* competition? It means one thing to a football player—who, at the final gun, is through for the day and will train for another week or two before the next game. It means something else to a baseball player, who may have another game the next day. It means something else yet to a swimmer—who, after finishing a race, may face another event in two hours.

The important considerations here, as in the previous section, are fluids and carbohydrates.

In multiple-event situations—swimming or wrestling, for example—nutrition between events is a real concern. If you compete in this kind of setting, you should begin your nutritional preparation for the next event as soon as your first event is over. The prescription is simple:

- Measure your bodyweight. For each pound of weight lost, drink 2 cups of water or a sports drink. Even when you consume fluids regularly during that exercise, you need this additional step to ensure complete rehydration afterward.

- If you have 90 minutes or more until your next event, try drinking a liquid meal preparation, but drink only about 250 to 500 calories' worth. That will restore a full range of nutrients—especially carbohydrates—to your body, and you will digest it quickly enough to avoid any discomfort when you resume exercising.

- If you have an hour or less until your next competition, eat a small, high-energy snack as soon as possible.

When your competition—regardless of the sport—is over for the day, your objective should be to resume normal training as quickly and efficiently as possible (or, if you have another competition the next day, to continue performing as efficiently as possible). To do this, you want to restore your body's fluid and energy reserves right away.

You need to do only two things:

- Follow the same rehydration guideline detailed above for multiple-event situations.
- Soon after competition, eat a high-carbohydrate meal.

If you were in good physical and nutritional shape prior to competition, you should be able to make the transition back to normal training without missing a beat.

❖   ❖   ❖

APPENDIX

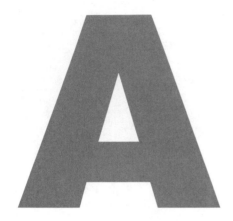

THE A.D.A. NUTRITIONAL RECOMMENDATIONS FOR ATHLETES

THE NUTRITIONAL DEMANDS OF ATHLETIC TRAINING

From time to time a paper appears whose information is so applicable and whose points are so clearly made that it justifies reprinting in full. This article, from the Journal of the American Dietetic Association, is such a paper. Reprinted with permission from the July, 1987 issue....

A proper, well-balanced diet is an essential component of any fitness or sports program. As more persons assume responsibility for their own health and fitness and engage in a variety of sports and exercise programs, it is essential that they have access to appropriate and accurate nutrition information. Those involved in more intense athletic activity require more specific information and education. This article addresses the needs of both groups and makes specific recommendations on how best to achieve their unique nutrition and fitness goals.

Position

It is the position of the *American Dietetic Association* to support the need for accurate and appropriate nutrition education to promote optimum fitness and well-being. The *American Dietetic Association* also recognizes the need for more specific nutrition recommendations for those individuals involved in more intense athletic activity.

DIETARY RECOMMENDATIONS FOR ADULT ATHLETES

CARBOHYDRATES

Current Average:	*45% of all calories*
Recommended Intake for Non-Athletes:	*50-60% of all calories (40-50% from complex carbs)*
Recommended Intake for Athletes:	*60-65% of all calories (50-55% from complex carbs)*
Recommended Intake for Endurance Athletes:	*65-70% of all calories (60-65% from complex carbs)*

PROTEIN

Current Average:	*1.5 grams/kilogram body weight per day*
Recommended Intake for Non-Athletes:	*0.8 gm/kg/day*
Recommended Intake for Athletes:	*1.0 gm/kg/day (12-15% of all calories)*
Recommended Intake for Endurance Athletes:	*1.0 gm/kg/day (12-15% of all calories)*

VITAMINS

VITAMINS	USRDA	RECOMMENDATION FOR ATHLETES
Vitamin A, IU*:	*5000*	*same*
Vitamin B_1 (thiamine), mg**:	*1.5*	*same*
Vitamin B_2 (riboflavin), mg:	*1.7*	*about 3.1*
Vitamin B_3 (niacin), mg:	*20*	*same*
Vitamin B_6 (pyridoxine), mg:	*2.0*	*same*
Vitamin B_{12} (cyanocobalamine), µg***:	*6.0*	*same*
Folic acid, mg:	*0.4*	*same*
Biotin, mg:	*0.3*	*same*
Pantothenic acid, mg:	*10*	*same*
Vitamin C (ascorbic acid), mg:	*60*	*same*
Vitamin D, IU:	*400*	*same*
Vitamin E, IU:	*30*	*same*

MINERALS

MINERALS	USRDA	RECOMMENDATION FOR ATHLETES
Calcium, mg:	*1000*	*if amenorrheic, may need 1500*
Chromium, µg:	*50-200*	*same*
Copper, mg:	*2*	*same*
Magnesium, mg:	*400*	*same*
Iron, mg:	*18*	*same*
Zinc, mg:	*15*	*same*
Selenium, µg:	*50-200*	*same*

*International Units   **milligrams   ***micrograms

Taking personal responsibility for one's health is a major force behind the fitness movement. Participants in exercise programs range from school-age children to adults of all ages, from elite competitors to weekend golfers. Although all these persons consider themselves athletes, their interests, skills, and training needs are varied. Messages from the marketplace on how best to achieve each of their unique nutrition and fitness goals can confuse the consumer.

There are several factors to consider when discussing appropriate nutrition for the athlete. Specific athletic events require different body composition for maximal performance. Body composition can be estimated indirectly by several methods, including anthropometric measurements, hydrostatic weighing, multiple isotope dilution, and electrical impedance units.

Energy demands are based on individual basal metabolic rate plus the intensity, duration, frequency, and type of activity involved. For weight reduction, a calorically prudent diet combined with appropriate exercise will increase the body's muscle mass while reducing body fat stores. Individuals engaged in vigorous exercise training programs may have energy needs ranging from 3000 to 6000 kcal [kilocalories] per day or more. Weight management, whether weight loss, gain, or maintenance, may be difficult to achieve without a well-planned dietary program.

Complex carbohydrates should account for at least 50% to 55% of total calories for the athlete. Carbohydrate loading will be beneficial only to athletes participating in long duration endurance or multiple-event competitions. It is now recommended that athletes follow a high-carbohydrate diet throughout training and begin a tapered rest approximately 7 days prior to the event, with complete rest the day before the event.

The current Recommended Dietary Allowance (RDA) of 0.8 gm protein per kilogram per day may be inadequate for endurance athletes. An intake of 1 gm/kg/day is advised, which is more than adequately met by the typical American diet. Excessive protein consumption has not been demonstrated to enhance athletic performance.

Extended physical activity may increase the need for some vitamins and minerals, which can easily be met by consuming a balanced diet in accordance with the extra caloric requirement. Although a nutritional deficiency can impair physical performance and cause several other detrimental effects, there is no conclusive evidence of performance enhancement with intakes in excess of the RDA. Consuming the RDA's for iron and calcium requires special attention by female athletes. Amenorrheic athletes may require additional calcium for calcium balance to accommodate both their lower estrogen levels and the decreased intestinal calcium absorption related to their prolonged training. Athletes may be at extra risk for developing iron deficiency because of sweat and intestinal losses, hematuria [blood in the urine], increased demands for total body hemoglobin, and poor dietary intakes. However, iron deficiency should not be confused with sports anemia, a condition defined as the increased destruction of erythrocytes [red blood cells] and a transient drop in hemoglobin as a result of an acute stress response to exercise; generally no supplement is required.

Proper hydration is essential for athletic performance. Dehydration can cause a reduction in maximal oxygen consumption and can compromise heat dissipation, which increases body temperature and results in a loss of coordination. Vigorous exercise blunts the thirst mechanism, making it difficult to replace fluid loss without a plan for periodic consumption. An adequate quantity of plain cool water will meet the fluid needs of most persons exercising in moderate climatic conditions. Extreme exercise levels and/or certain environmental conditions may warrant a low-dose supplemental electrolyte replacement beverage during endurance competitions to guard against electrolyte disturbances experienced as a result of excessive sweat loss.

Ergogenic aids are reputed to enhance performance above the levels anticipated under normal conditions. In most cases, they are without validation and are, in effect, more expensive forms of protein, sugars, or vitamins that provide psychological rather than proven physiological benefits. Alcohol has been shown to have no beneficial effect on exercise performance and, in fact, is more likely to impede performance. Caffeine, theorized to have a glycogen-sparing action during exercise, may offset fatigue, but its negative side effects may outweigh possible benefits.

What an athlete eats before competition makes a difference, both physically and psychologically. The pre-competition meal should be individualized to reflect different transit times, personal food preferences, and the scheduling of events to ensure gastric emptying and avoid discomfort or cramping. The meal should consist primarily of foods high in complex carbohydrates; foods high in fats and proteins that may require more time to digest should be avoided. The precompetition meal ought to be eaten 3½ to 4 hours prior to competition. A well-planned, balanced program is the basis for good health and enhanced athletic performance.

[Note: There is evidence that additional calcium alone for amenorrheic athletes is not sufficient to prevent osteoporosis. If you are amenorrheic, ask your doctor if you need supplemental estrogen as well.]

Journal of the American Dietetic Association
V 87 # 7: 933-9, July 1987

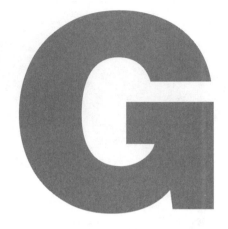

GLOSSARY

Aerobic: Literally, "with oxygen." For exercise, it describes the production of energy through the use of oxygen.

Alveoli: Terminal saclike dilations of the alveolar ducts in the lung. The extraction of oxygen from the air occurs in the alveoli.

Anaerobic: Literally, "without oxygen." For exercise, it describes the production of energy without oxygen.

ATP (adenosine triphosphate): A chemical compound that is the basis of all energy production within the human body. The breakdown of ATP molecules fuels every physiological process in the body.

Bronchii: Two large tubes through which air passes from the trachea into the lungs.

Bronchioles: Tube-like subdivisions of the two bronchii that carry air through the lungs to the alveoli.

Capillaries: The network of microscopic blood vessels that carries blood cells to the cells of body tissue.

Carbohydrate: A chemical compound composed of carbon and water whose main function is to serve as an energy fuel for the body. In the human body, carbohydrate is stored as glycogen in the muscle tissues and liver and as glucose in the blood.

Cardiac Output: The primary indicator of the functional capacity of the cardiovascular system. It is measured by stroke volume times frequency (heart rate).

Cardiovascular System: The continuous vascular circuit composed of the heart, lungs, and network of blood vessels that routes blood throughout the body.

CP (creatine phosphate): A chemical compound within the cells of the body that assists ATP in the production of energy for physiological functions.

Erythrocytes: Red blood cells that carry oxygen in the blood stream.

Free Fatty Acids: Chemical form of fat in the bloodstream that the body uses to produce energy.

Glucose: Simple form of carbohydrate in the blood that the body uses to produce ATP via both aerobic and anaerobic means.

Glycolysis: The transformation of cellular carbohydrate (glucose or glycogen) into energy-producing ATP.

Glycogen: Simple sugar form of carbohydrate that is stored within the muscles for use as energy.

Hemoglobin: A component of red blood cells that attaches itself to oxygen, thereby increasing the blood's oxygen-carrying capacity.

Lactate Threshold: The percentage of maximal oxygen uptake during exercise at which lactic acid production exceeds lactic acid clearing, resulting in the accumulation of lactate beyond a baseline level, negatively affecting aerobic performance.

Lactic Acid: By-product of anaerobic energy production that serves as an additional energy source but also halts energy production when excessive levels accumulate within the blood and muscles. Also known as *lactate*.

Mitochondria: A component of human muscle cells where ATP is produced.

Neurotransmitters: Chemical compounds that carry messages between brain cells.

OBLA (onset of blood lactate accumulation): see *Lactate Threshold*.

VO$_2$ Max: The largest volume of oxygen that your body can use during exercise.

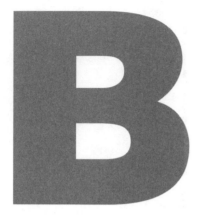

BIBLIOGRAPHY

TEXT SOURCES

Armstrong, R.B.; "Muscle fiber recruitment patterns and their metabolic correlates," in Horton, E.S. / Terjung, R.L. (eds), *Exercise, Nutrition, and Energy Metabolism*. Macmillan, New York, 1988.

Consolazio, C.F./Johnson, R./Pecora, L., *Physiological Measurement of Metabolic Function*. Mc-Graw Hill, New York, 1963.

Giese, A.C., *Cell Physiology*. W.B. Saunders, Philadelphia, 1979.

Gollnick, P.D. & Hermansen, L.; "Biomechanical adaptations to exercise. Anaerobic metabolism," in Wilmore, J.H. (ed), *Exercise and Sports Sciences Review*, Academic Press, New York, 1973.

Guyton, A.C., *Textbook of Medical Physiology*. Seventh Edition, W.B.Saunders, Philadelphia, 1986.

Hermansen, L.; "Effect of metabolic changes on force generation in skeletal muscle during maximal exercise," in *Human Muscle Fatigue: Physiological Mechanisms*. Pitman Medical, London, 1981.

Hermansen, L.; "Lactate production during exercise," in Pernow, B. / Saltin, B. (eds) *Muscle Metabolism During Exercise*, Plenum Press, New York, 1971.

Horton, E.S. / Terjung, R.L. (eds), *Exercise, Nutrition, and Energy Metabolism*. Macmillan, New York, 1988.

Jones, N.L. & Ehrsam, R.E.; "The Anaerobic Threshold," in Terjung, R.L. (ed), *Exercise and Sports Sciences Reviews*. Vol.10, Franklin Institute, Philadelphia, 1975.

Karlsson, J. & Jacobs, L. "Onset of blood lactate accumulation during exercise as a threshold concept. I. Theoretical considerations," *International Journal of Sports Medicine*. 1982;3:190.

Lehnigner, A.L., *Principles of Biochemistry*. Worth Publishers, New York, 1982.

Marieb, E.N., *Human Anatomy and Physiology*. Benjamin Cummings, Redwood City, 1989.

McArdle, W.D./Katch, F.I./Katch, V.L., *Exercise Physiology—Energy, Nutrition and Performance*, Third Edition, Lea and Febiger, Malvern, PA, 1991.

McArdle, W.D., et al.; "Specificity of run training on VO_2 max and heart rate changes during running and swimming," *Medicine and Sport Science*. 1978;10:16.

Rennie, D.W., et al.; "Energetics of swimming in man," in L.Lewille / J.Clarys, (eds.), *Swimming Illustrated*. University Park Press, Baltimore, 1975.

Saltin, B.; "Muscle fiber recruitment and metabolism in prolonged exhaustive dynamic exercise," in *Human Muscle Fatigue:Physiological Mechanisms*. Pitman Medical, London, 1981.

Sjödin, B., et al.; "The physiological background on onset blood lactate accumulation (OBLA)," in Komi, P.V.(ed.), *Proceedings of International Symposium of Sports Biology*, Champaign, IL, 1982.

Stryer, L., *Biochemistry*. Second Edition, McGraw-Hill, New York, 1985.

JOURNAL SOURCES

Acevedo, E.O. & Goldfarb, A.H.; "Increased training intensity effects on plasma lactate, ventilatory threshold, and endurance," *Medicine and Science in Sports and Exercise*. 1989;21:263.

Andrew, G.M., et al.; "Effect of athletic training on exercise cardiac output," *Journal of Applied Physiology*. 1966;21:603.

Bachman, J.C., & Horvath, S.M.; "Pulmonary function changes which accompany athletic training programs," *Research Quarterly*. 1968;39:235.

Barnard, R.J., et al.; "Cardiovascular responses to sudden strenuous exercise: heart rate, blood pressure, and ECG," *Journal of Applied Physiology.* 1973;34:883.

Basset, D.R., et al.; "Aerobic requirements of overground versus treadmill running," *Medicine and Science in Sports and Exercise.* 1985;17:477.

Belcastro, A.N. & Bonen, A.; "Lactic acid removal rates during controlled and uncontrolled recovery exercise," *Journal of Applied Physiology.* 1975;39:932.

Bender, P.R. & Martin, B.J.; "Maximal ventilation for exhausting exercise," *Medicine and Science in Sports and Exercise.* 1985;17:164.

Bergh, U., et al.; "Maximal oxygen uptake and muscle fiber types in trained and untrained humans," *Medicine and Sports Science.* 1978;10:151.

Brooks, G.A.; "Anaerobic threshold: review of the concept and directions for future research," *Medicine and Science in Sports and Exercise.* 1985;17:22.

Buno, M.J., et al.; "The effect of an acute bout of exercise on selected pulmonary function measurements," *Medicine and Science in Sports and Exercise.* 1981;13:290.

Burke, E.J. & Franks, B.D.; "Changes in VO$_2$ max resulting from bicycle training at different intensities holding total mechanical work constant," *Research Quarterly.* 1975;46:31.

Campbell, C.J., et al.; "Muscle fiber composition and performance capacities of women," *Medicine and Sports Science.* 1979;11:260.

Chasiotis, D.; "Role of Cyclic AMP and inorganic phosphate in the regulation of muscle glycogenolysis during exercise," *Medicine and Science in Sports and Exercise.* 1988;(20):545.

Christenson, E.H., et al.; "Intermittent and continuous running," *Acta Physiologica Scandinavica.* 1960;50:269.

Collander, E.B., et al.; "Blood pressure in resistance-trained athletes," *Canadian Journal of Sports Science.* 1988;13:31.

Conley, D.L., et al.; "Training for aerobic capacity and running economy," *Physician and Sportsmedicine.* 1981;9:107.

Costill, D.L.; "Metabolic responses during distance running," *Journal of Applied Physiology.* 1970;28:251.

Costill, D.L., et al.; "Fractional utilization of the aerobic capacity during distance running," *Medicine and Sports Science.* 1973;5:248.

Costill, D.L., et al.; "Glycogen depletion patterns in human muscle fibers during distance running," *Acta Physiologica Scandinavica*. 1973;89:374.

Costill, D.L., et al.; "Skeletal muscle enzyme and fiber composition in male and female track athletes," *Journal of Applied Physiology*. 1976;40:149.

Couldry, W.C., et al.; "Carotid vs. radial pulse counts," *Physician and Sportsmedicine*. 1982;10:67.

Cunningham, D.A. & Faulkner, J.A.; "The effect of training on aerobic and anaerobic metabolism during a short exhaustive run," *Medicine and Sports Science*. 1969;1:65.

Davies, K.J.A., et al.; "Biomechanical adaptation of mitochondria, muscle and whole-animal respiration to endurance training," *Archives of Biochemistry and Biophysics*. 1981;209:539.

Davis, J.A., et al.; "Anaerobic threshold alterations caused by endurance training in middle-aged men," *Journal of Applied Physiology*. 1979;46:1039.

Davis, J.A.; "Anaerobic threshold: review of the concept and directions for future research," *Medicine and Science in Sports and Exercise*. 1985;17:6.

Davis, J.A., et al.; "Anaerobic threshold and maximal aerobic power for three modes of exercise," *Journal of Applied Physiology*. 1976;41:544.

Dempsey, J.A.; "Is the lung built for exercise?," *Medicine and Science in Sports and Exercise*. 1986;18:143.

Donovan, C.M. & Brooks, G.A.; "Endurance training affects lactate clearance, not lactate production," *American Journal of Physiology*. 1983;83:244.

Eddy, D.O., et al.; "The effects of continuous and interval running in women and men," *European Journal of Applied Physiology*. 1977;37:83.

Essen, B., et al.; "Metabolic characteristics of fiber types in human skeletal muscles," *Acta Physiologica Scandinavica*. 1975;95:153.

Farrell, P.A., et al.; "Plasma lactate accumulation and distance running performance," *Medicine and Sports Science*. 1979;11:338.

Fellingham, G.W., et al.; "Calorie cost of walking and running," *Medicine and Sport Science*. 1978;10:132.

Fleck, S.J.; "Cardiovascular adaptations to resistance training," *Medicine and Science in Sports and Exercise*. 1988;20:S146.

Folinsbee, L.J., et al.; "Exercise respiratory pattern in elite cyclists and sedentary subjects," *Medicine and Science in Sports and Exercise.* 1983;15:503.

Fouriner, M., et al.; "Skeletal muscle adaptation in adolescent boys: sprint and endurance training and detraining," *Medicine and Science in Sports and Exercise.* 1982;14:453.

Fox, E.L., et al.; "Frequency and duration of interval training programs and changes in aerobic power," *Journal of Applied Physiology.* 1975;38:481.

Franklin, B.A.; "Aerobic exercise training programs for the upper body," *Medicine and Science in Sports and Exercise.* 1989;21:S141.

Fringer, M.N. & Stull, G.A.; "Changes in cardiorespiratory parameters during periods of training and detraining in young adult females," *Medicine and Sports Science.* 1974;6:20.

Gardner, G.W., et al.; "Use of carotid pulse for heart rate monitoring," *Medicine and Sports Science.* 1979;11:111.

Gaesser, G.A. & Rich, G.A.; "Effects of high- and low- intensity exercises on aerobic capacity and blood lipids," *Medicine and Science in Sports and Exercise.* 1984;16:269.

Gettman, L.R., et al.; "Specificity of arm training on aerobic power during swimming and running," *Medicine and Science in Sports and Exercise.* 1984;16:349.

Goldfinch, J., et al.; "Induced metabolic alkalosis and its effects on 400-m racing time," *European Journal of Applied Physiology.* 1988;57:45.

Gollnick, P., et al., "Effects of training on enzyme activity and fiber composition of human skeletal muscle," *Journal of Applied Physiology.* 1973;34:107.

Grimby, G., et al.; "Cardiac output during submaximal and maximal exercise in active middle-aged athletes," *Journal of Applied Physiology.* 1966;21:1150.

Grimby, G.; "Respiration in exercise," *Medicine and Sport Science.* 1969;1:9.

Henry, F.M.; "Aerobic oxygen consumption and alactic debt in muscular work," *Journal of Applied Physiology.* 1951;3:427.

Hagberg, J.M., et al.; "Effect of 12 months of intense exercise training on stroke volume in patients with coronary artery disease," *Circulation.* 1983;67:1194.

Hagberg, J.M., et al.; "Pulmonary function in young and older athletes and untrained men," *Journal of Applied Physiology.* 1988;65:101.

Henritze, J., et al.; "Effects of training at and above the lactate threshold and maximal oxygen uptake," *European Journal of Applied Physiology.* 1985;54:84.

Hickson, J.F./Wolinsky, I. (eds), *Nutrition in Exercise and Sports.* CRC Press, Boca Raton, FL, 1989.

Hickson, R.C., et al.; "Reduced training intensities and loss of aerobic power, endurance, and cardiac growth," *Journal of Applied Physiology.* 1985;58:492.

Hickson, R.C.; "Interference of strength development by simultaneously training for strength and endurance," *European Journal of Applied Physiology.* 1980;45:255.

Hickson, R.C., et al.; "Linear increase in aerobic power induced by a strenuous program of endurance exercise," *Journal of Applied Physiology.* 1977;42:373.

Hickson, R.C., et al.; "Reduced training duration effects on aerobic power, endurance and cardiac growth," *Journal of Applied Physiology.* 1982;53:255.

Houston, M.E. & Thompson, J.A.; "The response of endurance adapted adults to intense anaerobic training," *European Journal of Applied Physiology.* 1977;36:207.

Holloszy, J.O. & Coyle, E.F.; "Adaptations of skeletal muscle to endurance exercise and their metabolic consequences," *Journal of Applied Physiology.* 1984;56:834.

Howley, E.T., & Glover, M.E.; "The caloric cost of running and walking one mile for men and women," *Medicine and Sport Science.* 1974;6:235.

Ivy, J.L., et al.; "Muscle respiratory capacity and fiber type as determinants of lactate threshold," *Journal of Applied Physiology.* 1980;48:523.

Jacobs, I., et al.; "Onset of blood lactate accumulation during muscular exercise as a threshold concept," *Medicine and Science in Sports and Exercise.* 1987;19:368.

Jacobs, I.; "Blood lactate: implications for training and sports performance," *Sports Medicine.* 1986;3:10.

Jacobs, I.; "Sprint training effects on muscle myoglobin, enzymes, fiber types, and blood lactate," *Medicine and Science in Sports and Exercise.* 1987;19:368.

Karlsson, J., et al.; "Relevance of muscle fibers type to fatigue in short intense and prolonged exercise in man," in *Human Muscle Fatigue: Physiological Mechanisms*. Pitman Medical, London, 1981.

Karlsson, J.L., et al.; "Muscle lactate, ATP, and CP levels during exercise after physical training in man," *Journal of Applied Physiology*. 1972;33:199.

Katz, A., et al.; "Maximal exercise tolerance after induced alkalosis," *Journal of Sports Medicine*. 1984;5:107.

Katz, A. & Sahlin, K.; "Regulation of lactic acid production during exercise," *Journal of Applied Physiology*. 1988;65:509.

Kiyonaga, A., et al.; "Blood pressure and hormonal response to aerobic exercise," *Hypertension*. 1985;17:125.

Klein, J.P., et al.; "Hemoglobin affinity for oxygen during short-term exhaustive exercise," *Journal of Applied Physiology*. 1980;48:236.

Kumagi, S., et al.; "Relationship of the anaerobic threshold with the 5km, 10km, and 10 mile races," *European Journal of Applied Physiology*. 1982;49:13.

LaFontaine, T.P., et al.; "The maximal steady state versus selected running events," *Medicine and Science in Sports and Exercise*. 1981;13:190.

Lawrie, R.A.; "Effect of enforced exercise on myoglobin in muscle," *Nature*. 1953;171:1069.

Londeree, B.R. & Moeschberger, M.L.; "Effect of age and other factors on maximal heart rate," *Research Quarterly of Exercise and Sport*. 1982;53:297.

MacDougall, J.D., et al.; "Mitochondrial volume density in human skeletal muscle following heavy resistance training," *Medicine and Sports Science*. 1979;11:164.

Mainwood, G.W. & Renaud, J.M.; "The effect of acid-base on fatigue of skeletal muscle," *Canadian Journal of Physiology and Pharmacology*. 1985;(63)403.

Magel, J.R., et al.; "Specificity of swim training on maximum oxygen uptake," *Journal of Applied Physiology*. 1975;38:151.

Martin, B.J. & Stager, J.M.; "Ventilatory endurance in athletes and non-athletes," *Medicine and Science in Sports and Exercise*. 1981;13:21.

McArdle, W.D., et al.; "Comparison of continuous and discontinuous treadmill and bicycle tests for VO$_2$max," *Medicine and Sport Science*. 1973;5:156.

McLellan, T.M. & Skinner, J.S. "Blood lactate removal during active recovery related to aerobic threshold," *International Journal of Sports Medicine.* 1982;3:224.

Miles, D.S.; "Cardiovascular responses to upper body exercise in normals and cardiac patients," *Medicine and Science in Sports and Exercise.* 1989;21:S126.

Minotti, J.R., et al.; "Training-induced skeletal muscle adaptations are independent of systemic adaptations," *Journal of Applied Physiology.* 1990;68:289.

Pendergast, D.R.; "Cardiovascular, respiratory, and metabolic responses to upper body exercise," *Medicine and Science in Sports and Exercise.* 1989;21:S121.

Pernow, B. & Karlsson, J.; "Muscle ATP, CP and lactate in submaximal and maximal exercise," in Pernow, B. / Saltin, B., (eds), *Muscle Metabolism During Exercise.* Plenum Press, New York, 1971.

Pollock, M.L., et al.; "Effects of mode of training on cardiovascular function and body composition of adult men," *Medicine and Sports Science.* 1975;7:139.

Rand, P.W., et al.; "Influence of athletic training on hemoglobin-oxygen affinity," *American Journal of Physiology.* 1973;224:1334.

Saltin, B.; "Physiological effects of physical conditioning," *Medicine and Sports Science.* 1969;1:50.

Scheuer, J. & Tipton, C.M.; "Cardiovascular adaptations to physical training," *Annual Review of Physiology.* 1977;39:221.

Sedlock, D.A., et al.; "Accuracy of subject-palpitated carotid pulse after exercise," *Physician and Sportsmedicine.* 1983;11:106.

Sharkey, B.J.; "Intensity and duration of training and the development of cardiorespiratory endurance," *Medicine and Sports Science.* 1970;2:197.

Simoneau, J.A., et al.; "Human skeletal muscle fiber type alteration with high-intensity intermittent training," *European Journal of Applied Physiology.* 1985;54:240.

Stubbing, D.C., et al.; "Pulmonary mechanics during exercise in normal males," *Journal of Applied Physiology.* 1980;49:506.

Tanaka, K., et al.; "Relationship of anaerobic threshold and onset of blood lactate accumulation with endurance performance," *European Journal of Applied Physiology.* 1983;52:51.

Tanaka, K., et al.; "A longitudinal assessment of anaerobic threshold and distance-running performance," *Medicine and Science in Sports and Exercise.* 1984;16:278.

Taylor, D.J., et al.; "Energetics of human muscle: exercise- induced ATP depletion," *Magnetic Resonance Medicine.* 1986;3:44.

Terjung, R.I., et al.; "Cardiovascular adaptation to twelve minutes of mild daily exercise in middle-aged sedentary men," *Journal of the American Geriatric Society.* 1973;21:164.

Tesch, P.A. & Karlsson, J.; "Muscle fiber type and size in untrained muscles of elite athletes," *Journal of Applied Physiology.* 1985;59:1716.

Tesch, P.A. & Larsson, L.; "Muscle hypertrophy in bodybuilders," *European Journal of Applied Physiology.* 1982;49:301.

Toner, M.M., et al.; "Cardiovascular adjustment to exercise distributed between the upper and lower body," *Medicine and Science in Sports and Exercise.* 1990;22:773.

Wasserman, K., et al.; "Anaerobic threshold and respiratory gas exchange during exercise," *Journal of Applied Physiology.* 1973;35:236.

Weltman, A.; "The lactate threshold and endurance performance," *Advances in Sports Medicine and Fitness.* 1989;2:91.

Whipp, B.J. & Wasserman, K.; "The effect of work intensity on the transient respiratory response immediately following exercise," *Medicine and Sports Science.* 1973;5:14.

Yoshida, T., et al.; "Blood lactate parameters related to aerobic capacity and endurance performance," *European Journal of Applied Physiology.* 1987;56:7.

❖ ❖ ❖

Index

SynerStretch: For Total Body Flexibility...FAST!

Two programs in one: Both deliver lower- and upper-body flexibility in less than 8 minutes a day! **Syner-Stretch A** is for you if you need to maintain your flexibility. Originally designed for martial artists—who depend on extreme flexibility— **SynerStretch A** will also help bodybuilders, dancers, and other athletes stay flexible in less than *5 minutes per workout*. A great way to end a training session of any kind! **SynerStretch B** is for you if you need to increase your flexibility. Not only does it take less than 8 minutes, but because it makes use of a new, relatively unknown technique (Isometric Agonist Contraction/Relaxation), it eliminates most of the pain usually associated with stretching. It works! When you order **SynerStretch**, you get both programs in one manual. *Get loose, and stay loose with **SynerStretch**. A 28 p. illustrated manual.* **Also available on video.**

Power ForeArms!

Here at last is a program that specifically targets the hard-to-develop forearm muscles. Like all Health For Life programs, **Power ForeArms!** is based on the Synergism principle and yields maximum results in minimum time. Designed for serious bodybuilders and martial artists, **Power ForeArms!** will help you build strong, solid, massive forearms in just 7 to 12 minutes, twice a week. Give **Power ForeArms!** a try. *A 32 p. illustrated manual.* **Also available on video.**

SynerShape: A Scientific Weight Loss Guide

We're surrounded by weight loss myths. Crash diets. Spot reducing. Exotic herbs. Still, most plans fail, and most people who lose weight gain it back again. Is there really an honest, effective solution? **Yes! Syner-Shape** represents the next generation in awareness of how the body gains and metabolizes fat. It synthesizes the most recent findings on nutrition, exercise, and psychology into a TOTAL program, offering you the tools you need to shape the body you want. **SynerShape** works. Let it work for *you! A 24 p. illustrated manual.*

The Psychology of Weight Loss

This special program-on-tape picks up where **SynerShape** leaves off. Noted psychologist Carol Landesman explores eating problems and *solutions* based on the latest research into human behavior and metabolism. Then, through a series of exercises, she helps you begin to heal the emotional conflicts behind your weight problem. **The Psychology of Weight Loss** is a unique program that brings the power of the therapy process into the privacy of your home. *A 90-minute guided introspection. On audio cassette.*

The 7-Minute Rotator Cuff Solution

Almost everyone who works out experiences some kind of rotator cuff injury during a lifetime of training. Any of these injuries could spell the end of a workout career, but most can be prevented. **The 7-Minute Rotator Cuff Solution** is a quick, simple program to help prevent (or help you recover from) rotator cuff injuries. It details how the shoulder works, what can go wrong and why, and exactly what to do (and not do) to stop shoulder problems before they happen. Plus: a simple 7-minute exercise program that can eliminate shoulder pain and restore normal shoulder function in just a few weeks. *144 pp., illustrated.*

For price and order information, or
to receive a FREE copy of the Health For Life Catalogue
call 1-800-874-5339
or write us at...

Health For Life
Suite 483, 8033 Sunset Blvd.
Los Angeles, CA 90046-2427